Contents

Osteopathic and Chiropractic Techniques for the Foot and Ankle

by the same author

Dry Needling for Manual Therapists
*Points, Techniques and Treatments, Including Electroacupuncture
and Advanced Tendon Techniques*
Giles Gyer, Jimmy Michael and Ben Tolson
ISBN 978 1 84819 255 3
eISBN 978 0 85701 202 9

Osteopathic and Chiropractic Techniques for Manual Therapists
A Comprehensive Guide to Spinal and Peripheral Manipulations
Jimmy Michael, Giles Gyer and Ricky Davis
ISBN 978 1 84819 326 0
eISBN 978 0 85701 281 4

Advanced Osteopathic and Chiropractic Techniques for Manual Therapists
Adaptive Clinical Skills for Peripheral and Extremity Manipulation
Giles Gyer and Jimmy Michael
ISBN 978 0 85701 394 1
eISBN 978 0 85701 395 8

Spine and Joint Articulation for Manual Therapists
Giles Gyer, Jimmy Michael and Ben Calvert
ISBN 978 1 90914 131 5
eISBN 978 1 91208 518 7

OSTEOPATHIC AND CHIROPRACTIC TECHNIQUES FOR THE FOOT AND ANKLE

*Clinical Understanding and Advanced Treatment Applications
and Rehabilitation for Manual Therapists*

Giles Gyer and Jimmy Michael
with Dr Kumar Kunasingam

SINGING DRAGON

LONDON AND PHILADELPHIA

First published in Great Britain in 2023 by Singing Dragon, an imprint of Jessica Kingsley Publishers
An imprint of Hodder & Stoughton Ltd
An Hachette UK Company

1

Disclaimer: The information contained in this book is not intended to replace the services of trained medical professionals or to be a substitute for medical advice. The complementary therapy described in this book may not be suitable for everyone to follow. You are advised to consult a doctor before embarking on any complementary therapy programme and on any matters relating to your health, and in particular on any matters that may require diagnosis or medical attention.

A CIP catalogue record for this title is available from the British Library and the Library of Congress

ISBN 978 1 83997 201 0
eISBN 978 1 83997 202 7

Printed and bound in China by Leo Paper Products Ltd

Jessica Kingsley Publishers' policy is to use papers that are natural, renewable and recyclable products and made from wood grown in sustainable forests. The logging and manufacturing processes are expected to conform to the environmental regulations of the country of origin.

Singing Dragon
Carmelite House
50 Victoria Embankment
London EC4Y 0DZ

www.singingdragon.com

Disclaimer

To the fullest extent of the law, neither the publisher nor the authors assume any liability for any injury and/or damage to persons or property incurred as a result of the instructions or ideas contained in the material herein. This field is constantly evolving as new research and experience broaden our knowledge. As a result, changes in professional practice may be necessary. Therapists and researchers should rely on their own expertise in evaluating and using any information included in this book. They should be mindful of their own safety as well as the safety of others in their care. With respect to any techniques identified, readers are advised to research the most current information available on procedures, dosage, method and duration of treatment, and contraindications. It is the responsibility of the therapist to provide the appropriate treatment for their patients, taking into account all the necessary safety precautions.

Acknowledgements

With special thanks to the following clinicians, whose help and contributions to this text have been invaluable:

Dr James Inklebarger, MD, London, UK

Dr Kumar Kunasingam, consultant orthopaedic surgeon, BSc (Hons), MBBS (Eng), MRCS (Eng), FRCS (Tr&Orth), DipSEM & DipOrth

Iain Barrowman, BSc (Hons) – Physiotherapy, CSCS & ASCC

We would like to thank Dr Kunasingam for his time and knowledge in helping to put this project together; working together as therapists and doctors to help create better clinical outcomes for patients is the key and requires teamwork, understanding and leaving the ego at the door.

Chapter 1

Understanding the Foot and Ankle

Healthy ankles and feet are vital for our mobility and independence. These two structures of our body work together as a functional unit to coordinate movements of gait, transfer total body weight and withstand forces during propulsion. These activities, however, make them highly susceptible to trauma and static deformities, which may ultimately lead to injury, overloading, chronic disability and potentially surgical interventions.

The burden of ankle and foot problems encountered by primary physicians is not insubstantial. This was demonstrated in a recent population-based study where the authors analysed data from the UK Clinical Practice Research Datalink (Ferguson *et al.*, 2019). They reported that the prevalence of foot and ankle pain in the UK population of all ages is about 3% (2980 per 100,000), and females are more commonly affected than males (54.4% and 45.6%, respectively). The study also reported around 34,000 referrals to physiotherapists during the period (2010–2013). These estimates, however, are found to be much higher for the older population (≥ 45 years). In fact, a systematic review reported a pooled prevalence estimate of 24% and 15% for foot pain and ankle pain, respectively (Thomas *et al.*, 2011).

Foot and ankle conditions are a common presentation in clinical practice. They may make up a substantial number of all visits in manual therapy clinics, and issues within the foot and ankle can be linked to other presenting conditions such as knee, hip and lower back complaints. Hence, a solid understanding of foot and ankle anatomy is essential for correct diagnosis and treatment. Having a good grasp of their underlying structures is like having a road map to navigate various parts of the foot and ankle. In fact, most structures in this region (e.g. bones, joints, tendons) are easily palpable and tend to show symptoms just where they are affected.

This book presents the most recent knowledge on foot and ankle pathology, physical and clinical diagnosis and non-invasive and invasive treatment options, giving therapists a selection of options to access within the clinic. We emphasise that prevention is better than cure, so a structured rehabilitation process and good treatment protocols can be beneficial in avoiding invasive procedures. In this chapter, we briefly overview the various anatomic structures of the foot and ankle and how they work together.

Basic anatomy

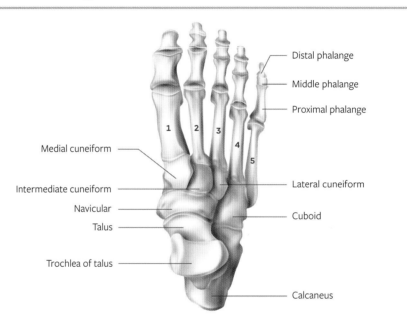

Figure 1.1 Anterior foot anatomy

In the appendicular skeleton, the most distal parts of the lower limb are the ankle and foot. These two structures form a highly complex system made up of bones, joints, ligaments and tendons, supported by intrinsic and extrinsic muscles. All of these structures work together in perfect coordination like a finely tuned machine and serve the body with various important functions (Bonnel *et al.*, 1998; Ficke and Byerly, 2020). These include:

- coordinating movements of gait

- providing balance to stand upright

- allowing flexibility to adapt to uneven surfaces

- ensuring a high degree of stability to perform diverse activities of daily living

- supporting varying degrees of weight-bearing

- absorbing shocks of excessive forces while running, jumping or climbing.

The ankle

The ankle joint is the junction where the lower leg and foot meet. It is the result of the articulation of three bones: the tibia, the fibula and the talus. The articulation brings the dome of the talus in contact with the recess formed by the distal tibia and fibula (Brockett and Chapman, 2016).

In medical terminology, the term 'ankle' refers specifically to the talocrural joint. However, in common usage, it often refers to the region or angle between the foot and leg (Moore *et al.*, 2013; Manganaro *et al.*, 2019). Owing to the strong bony and ligamentous structures, the ankle joint functions with a high degree of stability and can withstand high compressive and shear forces (Brockett and Chapman, 2016). It allows dorsiflexion and plantarflexion movements of the foot.

Ankle joints

The joints of the ankle and foot are unlike many other joints in the body. They work in an 'as needed' manner and can exhibit both static and dynamic activities. The ankle includes three joints: the talocrural joint, the subtalar joint and the inferior tibiofibular joint (Bonnel *et al.*, 1998).

The talocrural joint

- It is a synovial hinge joint that joins the dome of the talus with the distal tibia-fibula.

- Also known as the tibiotalar joint.

- It permits dorsiflexion and plantarflexion movements via axis in talus.

Note: The talocrural is the only joint in the human body joined in a mortise and tenon manner. The tibia and fibula connect with each other via tibiofibular ligaments, forming a concave surface, or mortise, that connects with the talar dome distally (Brockett and Chapman, 2016).

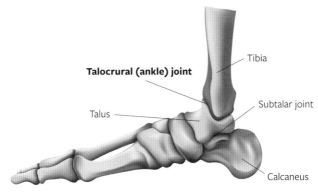

Figure 1.2 The talocrural joint

The subtalar joint

- The subtalar joint, also called the talocalcaneal joint, is formed between two of the tarsal bones: the talus and the calcaneus (heel bone).

- It is a modified multiaxial joint located within the hindfoot, just below the talocrural joint.

- It involves three articulations between the talus and the calcaneus: anterior, middle and posterior.

- It permits inversion and eversion motions of the ankle and hindfoot.

- It also allows slight rotational motions between the foot and the lower leg within frontal and horizontal planes, without involving the heel bone (Krähenbühl *et al.*, 2017).

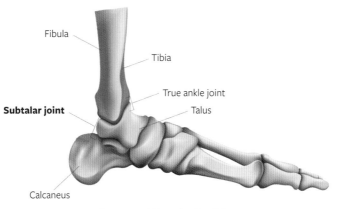

Figure 1.3 The subtalar joint

Inferior tibiofibular joint

- The inferior (distal) tibiofibular joint is a syndesmosis formed by joining the distal end of the fibula with the lateral side of the tibia (Mróz *et al.*, 2015).

- The syndesmosis is strengthened by tough fibrous bands – the interosseus ligament and the tibiofibular ligaments (anterior, posterior and transverse).

- The joint primarily plays a stabilising role to help maintain ankle joint integrity. It also permits slight movements to allow the lateral malleolus to rotate laterally when the ankle dorsiflexes.

- The joint is highly susceptible to injuries due to its ligamentous constraint. Eversion injuries and ankle fractures often affect this joint (Clanton and Paul, 2002).

Ankle ligaments

The ligaments surrounding the ankle can be broadly divided into two systems: the lateral and the medial ligamentous complex (Bonnel *et al.*, 1998).

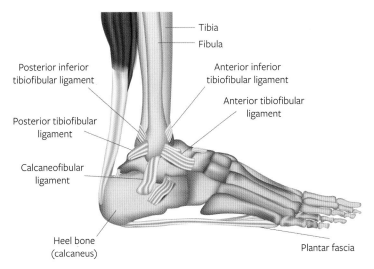

Figure 1.4 Lateral ankle ligaments

The lateral collateral complex includes three separate ligaments:

- anterior talofibular ligament

- posterior talofibular ligament

- calcaneofibular ligament.

The anterior and posterior talofibular ligaments connect the talus to the fibula. The calcaneofibular ligament attaches the fibula to the calcaneus.

The medial collateral ligaments consist of two layers: superficial and deep.

The superficial layer, also called the deltoid ligament, includes four ligaments:

- the anterior tibiotalar ligament

- the posterior tibiotalar ligament

- the tibionavicular ligament

- the tibiocalcaneal ligament.

These four ligaments connect the tibia to the talus, the navicular and the calcaneus, forming a triangle-like shape (Golanó *et al.*, 2010).

The deep layer includes two ligaments: the deep anterior tibiotalar ligament and the deep posterior tibiotalar ligament.

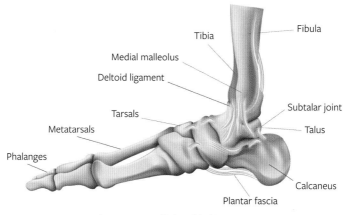

Figure 1.5 Medial ankle ligaments

The foot

The foot is a biomechanically complex structure located distal to the ankle joint. It consists of many anatomic structures (e.g. bones, joints, ligaments, muscles) that all work together to coordinate movements of gait, support the body weight, allow for locomotion, withstand forces during propulsion and transfer ground reaction forces (Manganaro *et al.*, 2019; Ficke and Byerly, 2020).

Bony anatomy

There are 26 bones in each foot, which can be divided into three groups: the tarsal bones (7), the metatarsal bones (5) and the phalanges (14). These bones form a series of arches in the foot (Tang and Bordoni, 2021).

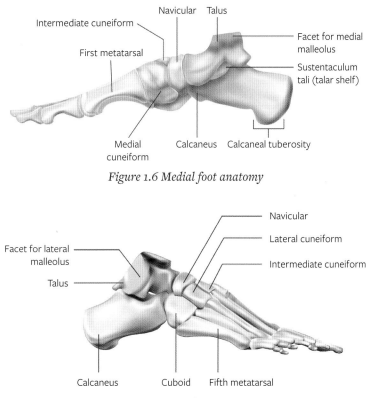

Figure 1.6 Medial foot anatomy

Figure 1.7 Lateral foot anatomy

The tarsal bones, also called the tarsus, are a cluster of seven articulating bones that form the posterior half of the foot. These include the talus, the calcaneus, the navicular, the cuboid and the three cuneiforms (medial, intermediate and lateral).

- **The talus** is the most superior of the tarsal bones. It forms the ankle joint, articulating with the distal tibia and fibula.

- **The calcaneus** is the largest bone of the foot. It forms the heel and serves as the attachment site for the large calf muscles.

- **The navicular** is a small bone located in front of the talus. It articulates posteriorly with the talus and anteriorly with the three cuneiforms.

- **The cuboid** is a square-shaped bone located at the anterior end of the calcaneus. It articulates posteriorly with the calcaneus and medially with the navicular and the lateral cuneiform.

- **The cuneiforms** are wedge-shaped bones with an extensive superior surface but a narrow inferior surface.

The metatarsal bones, also known as the metatarsus, are a group of five elongated bones (numbered 1–5) that form the anterior half of the foot. These bones are located between the tarsus and the phalanges. The second of these bones is the longest of all, whereas the first is thicker and shortest.

The phalanges include a total of 14 phalanx bones distributed in five toes (numbered 1–5). Four of these toes contain three phalanx bones: proximal, middle and distal phalanges. The hallux is analogous to the thumb, with two phalanx bones: the proximal and distal phalanges (Standring, 2008; Khan and Varacallo, 2019).

Subdivision of the foot

Structurally, the foot can be subdivided into three main parts: the hindfoot, the midfoot and the forefoot.

- **The hindfoot** is the region closest to the centre of the body. It contains two of the seven tarsal bones (the talus and the calcaneus).

- **The midfoot** is made up of the remaining five tarsal bones: the three cuneiforms, the cuboid and the navicular. The midtarsal joint separates the midfoot from the hindfoot. It constitutes the arches of the foot and works as a shock absorber.

- **The forefoot** contains the five metatarsals, the respective phalanges and associated soft-tissue structures. The tarsometatarsal joint, or the Lisfranc joint, separates it from the midfoot (Standring, 2008).

Foot joints

The foot includes a total of 33 joints, which help accommodate the stability and mobility functions. These joints form wherever two or more of the foot bones connect (Tate, 2009; Card and Bordoni, 2019). Below are some of the most important joints of the foot.

Intertarsal joints

The intertarsal joints are the articulations between the seven tarsal bones of the foot. These joints include:

- the subtalar joint (see 'Ankle joints')

- the talocalcaneonavicular joint (see below)

- the calcaneocuboid joint (see below)

- the cuneonavicular joint – formed between the navicular and the three cuneiforms

- the cuboideonavicular joint – formed between the navicular and the cuboid

- the intercuneiform joint – joints among the three cuneiform bones.

Midtarsal joint

- Also known as transverse tarsal joint (or Chopart's joint).

- It combines the junction between the hindfoot and the midfoot and includes two joints:

    o The talonavicular joint is formed between the talus and navicular. It is the most anterior part of the talocalcaneonavicular joint.

    o The calcaneocuboid joint is formed between the calcaneus and the cuboid (Tweed *et al.*, 2008).

Talocalcaneonavicular joint

- A compound, multiaxial joint – the rounded head of the talus articulates with the navicular and the calcaneus.

- It includes two articulations: an anterior talocalcaneal articulation and a talonavicular articulation.

Tarsometatarsal joint complex

- Arthrodial joints formed between the tarsal bones of the midfoot (the three cuneiform bones and the cuboid bone) and the bases of the metatarsal bones.

- Strong interosseus dorsal and plantar ligaments strengthen this joint complex.

Intermetatarsal joints

- Synovial joints that involve articulations between the bases of the second to fifth metatarsal bones.

- Serve to uphold the lateral stability of the forefoot.

Metatarsophalangeal joints

- Ellipsoid joints formed by joining the heads of the metatarsal bones with the bases of the proximal bones (proximal phalanges).

Interphalangeal joints

- Ginglymoid (hinge) joints formed by the articulations between the superior surfaces on the phalangeal heads and the adjacent phalangeal bases.

- Subdivide into two sets of articulations: proximal and distal interphalangeal joints.

- Each toe contains two interphalangeal joints, except for the hallux, which has only one (Ficke and Byerly, 2020).

Muscles of the ankle and foot

The ankle and foot consist of 31 muscles, which are connected to the osseous structures by the tendons. These muscles primarily assist in the coordinated movements of the ankle and foot structures. They also play a secondary role to ensure osseous and ligamentous stability (Brockett and Chapman, 2016; Card and Bordoni, 2019).

The muscles of the ankle and foot can be classified into two groups: the extrinsic muscles and the intrinsic muscles (31 total – 12 extrinsic and 19 intrinsic). The extrinsic muscles arise from the leg skeleton and insert within the foot. They are organised by four compartments (see Table 1.1).

The intrinsic muscles originate and insert within the foot. They can be divided into two groups: the dorsal group and the plantar (sole) group. The dorsal aspect contains only two intrinsic muscles – the extensor digitorum brevis and the extensor hallucis brevis. The plantar aspect consists of the remaining intrinsic muscles, including the abductor hallucis, the flexor hallucis brevis, the quadratus plantae, flexor digitorum brevis, the lumbricals, digiti minimi, flexor digiti minimi, and the dorsal and plantar interossei. These muscles primarily function to support and control the movements of the toes (Bonnel *et al.*, 1998; Manganaro *et al.*, 2019).

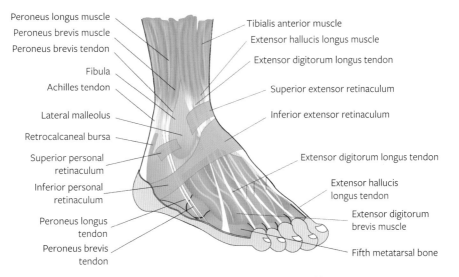

Figure 1.8 Muscles of the foot and ankle

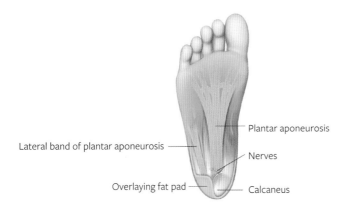

Figure 1.9 Plantar fascia

Table 1.1 The extrinsic muscles of the ankle and foot

Compartment name	Muscles	Movement
Anterior compartment (4 muscles)	Extensor digitorum longus Extensor hallucis longus muscles Tibialis anterior Peroneus (or fibularis) tertius	Dorsiflexion, eversion and inversion
Lateral compartment (2 muscles)	Peroneus brevis Peroneus longus	Plantarflexion and eversion
Posterior compartment (3 muscles)	Gastrocnemius Soleus Plantaris	Plantarflexion
Deep posterior compartment (3 muscles)	Flexor hallucis longus Flexor digitorum longus Tibialis posterior	Plantarflexion and inversion

Sources: Manganaro et al. (2019); Tang and Bordoni (2021)

Joints of the knee, ankle and foot

The knee joint is a bicompartmental synovial joint in human anatomy and is the largest in the human body. The joint occurs between the femur and the tibia bones. The joint also includes articulation between the patella and femur. The tibia and fibula articulate with each other at the superior and inferior tibio-fibular joints. All bones of the knee except the fibula play a role in movement (Standring, 2016).

Inferior to the knee joint is the talocrural joint (ankle joint). This joint is formed by the distal ends of the tibia and fibula 'gripping' the talus. Within the foot there are multiple joints that may be classified topographically based on whether they are in the hindfoot, midfoot or forefoot. These joints perform the various complex movements required as the foot fulfils its functional roles as a platform for standing and for shock absorption and propulsion in gait (Magee *et al.*, 2016).

Table 1.2 The joints of the knee, ankle and foot

Joint name	Description	Function
Knee joint	A bicompartmental synovial (modified hinge) joint Forms a complex hinge between three bones: the femur, the tibia and the patella Consists of different joints: tibiofemoral – between tibia and femur; patellofemoral joint – between femur; and the superior tibiofibular joint – between tibia and fibula Enclosed by a single articular capsule that enfolds the entire joint complex	Allows flexion and extension of the leg Ensures weight-bearing support of the body Allows transmission of body weight in vertical and horizontal directions Superior tibiofibular joint allows slight gliding motion Tolerates minor degree of internal and external rotation when flexed
Tibiofemoral joint	A modified hinge synovial joint Connects between the medial and the lateral condyles of the femur and the tibial condyles of the tibia Reinforced by two wedge-shaped articular discs: the medial meniscus and lateral meniscus	Assists as the weight-bearing joint of the knee Permits flexion and extension of the leg Allows some medial and lateral rotation of the leg
Patellofemoral joint	A diarthrodial plane joint Articulates the anterior and distal part of the femur with the patella (kneecap) Consists of the posterior surface of the patella and the trochlear surface of the distal anterior femur	Provides stability and strength to the knee joint Conveys tensile forces generated by the quadriceps to the patellar tendon Increases lever arm of the extensor mechanism Permits the knee to straighten when standing Helps to perform the activities of daily living (walking, cycling, stair climbing, jogging and squatting)
Proximal tibiofibular joint	A diarthrodial plane joint between the medial facet of the head of the fibula and the tibial facet on the posterolateral tibial condyle Has a fibrous capsule strengthened by anterior and posterior superior tibiofibular ligaments and tendinous insertions, making it intrinsically stable when the knee is stretched	Allows twisting movements of the leg Disperses torsional stresses applied at the ankle Transfers load between the feet and the body Dissipates lateral tibial bending movements

Joint name	Description	Function
Distal tibiofibular joint	A syndesmotic joint Formed by joining the distal end of the fibula with the lateral side of the tibia Is supported by strong interosseus ligament	The inferior segment assists in stabilising the tibiofibular syndesmosis Permits slight movements for the lateral malleolus to rotate laterally when the ankle dorsiflexes Helps to uphold the ankle joint integrity
Ankle or talocrural joint	A hinge joint between the distal ends of tibia and fibula and the trochlea of the talus Is reinforced by strong ligamentous structures that provide stability to the ankle Surrounded by a loose connective tissue called paratenon Joint is maintained by the shape of the talus and its tight fit between the tibia and fibula. In the neutral position	Facilitates rotation about an axis of rotation Permits dorsiflexion and plantarflexion movements via axis in talus
Subtalar or talocalcaneal joint	A joint formed by two bones in the foot: the talus and the calcaneus (heel bone) Includes three articulations between talus and calcaneus: anterior, middle and posterior	Allows internal and external rotation of the foot
Talocalcaneonavicular joint	A joint between the navicular, talus and calcaneus bones Comprises two articulations: a frontal talocalcaneal and a talonavicular	Allows pronation and supination of the foot
Calcaneocuboid joint	A joint formed between the calcaneus and the cuboid bone Strengthened by bifurcate, long plantar and plantar calcaneocuboid ligaments	Allows minor gliding movements between the calcaneus and the cuboid bone
Tarsometatarsal or Lisfranc joints	Arthrodial joints Formed between the bones of the second row of the tarsus and the bases of the metatarsal bones Joints are stabilised by strong interosseus dorsal and plantar ligaments	Allow small gliding movements at the feet

Intermetatarsal joints	Robust synovial joints Involve articulations between the bases of the second to fifth metatarsal bones Interosseus dorsal and plantar ligaments provide strength	Allow slight gliding movements at the feet
Metatarsophalangeal joints	Ovoid joints formed between the heads of the metatarsal bones and the bases of the proximal phalanges Reinforced by collateral, deep transverse metatarsal and plantar ligaments	Permit a variety of movements at the toes, including flexion, extension, abduction, adduction and circumduction
Interphalangeal joints	Ginglymoid (hinge) joints Articulations between the phalanges of the toes Subdivided into two sets of articulations: proximal interphalangeal joints and distal interphalangeal joints	Allows limited flexion and extension of the medial and distal phalanges

Sources: Norkin and White (2009); Magee et al. (2016); Standring (2016); Giangarra and Manske (2018)

Range of motion

Ankle

The ankle is a hinge joint between the distal ends of tibia and fibula and the trochlea of the talus. The joint enables rotation about an axis of rotation and permits dorsiflexion and plantarflexion movements via axis in talus (Young *et al.*, 2013).

Table 1.3 Approximate range of motion of the ankle

Movement type	Range of motion (degrees)
Normal dorsiflexion	0–50
Normal plantarflexion	0–20
Dorsiflexion, knee extended	14–48
Dorsiflexion, knee flexed	16–60

Source: Brockett and Chapman (2016)

Foot

The foot is divided into three parts, namely hindfoot, midfoot and forefoot. It functions to support body weight, provide balance, absorb shock and transfer ground reaction forces. Various joints are found on the foot including talocrural, subtalar, midtarsal, tarsometatarsal, metatarsophalangeal and interphalangeal joints. The joints display different types of motion. The talocrural joint allows for dorsiflexion and plantarflexion movements in the sagittal plane, while the subtalar joint permits pronation and supination movements. The midtarsal joint allows inversion and eversion, and flexion and extension. The metatarsophalangeal provides motion in the sagittal and transverse planes with flexion, extension, adduction and abduction motions. The interphalangeal joints allow motion in the sagittal plane, allowing pure flexion and extension (Brockett and Chapman, 2016).

Table 1.4 Range of motion of the foot joints

Joint name	Movement type	Range of motion (degrees)
Subtalar joint	Inversion	0–50
	Eversion	0–26
Metatarsophalangeal joints	Flexion (hallux)	0–45
	Extension (hallux)	0–80
	Flexion (lesser toes)	0–40
	Extension (lesser toes)	0–70
Interphalangeal joints	Flexion (hallux)	0–90
	Flexion (lesser toes)	0–30
	Extension (hallux and other toes)	0–80

Sources: Oatis (1988); Blackwood et al. (2005); Norkin and White (2009)

Common injuries

Injuries to the knee, ankle and foot are among the most frequent musculoskeletal injuries occurring in all demographic groups. These injuries are often attributed to trauma resulting from sporting accidents, falling from height, road traffic accidents and violent activity, to name but a few. Due to frequent overuse of the lower extremity in sporting activities, athletes often injure their ankles, feet or knees, and this may result in short-term or long-term disability leading to potential loss of productivity and income. The most common injuries of the knee, ankle and foot are summarised in Table 1.5.

Table 1.5 Common injuries of the knee, ankle and foot

Common injuries	Incidence	Characteristics
Anterior cruciate ligament sprain	68.6 per 100,000 person-years (US) 8.06 per 100,000 person-years (UK)	A very frequent knee injury The anterior cruciate ligament is torn, usually with a 'pop' – resulting in knee instability Higher incidence in athletes participating in sports such as American football, soccer, tennis, downhill skiing, volleyball and basketball that put a lot of strain on the knees Associated with sudden directional changes of the lower extremity, or sudden stops from running May also occur with high load landing from a jump Half of these injuries may result in damage to other knee structures (i.e. meniscus, articular cartilage, other ligaments)
Medial collateral ligament sprain	24 per 100,000 person-years (US) 5.21 per 100,000 person-years (UK)	Another high-frequency knee injury The medial collateral ligament which prevents the knee from bending inward is torn Frequently associated with athletes in contact sports (e.g. American football, rugby, wrestling, judo, rugby, hockey) Often occurs due to a hit or direct blow to the outer aspect of the knee Usually occurs after rapid directional changes while running as well as bending or twisting the lower extremity May include a 'popping' noise accompanied by pain, swelling and tenderness around the knee
Meniscal tear	61 per 100,000 person-years (US) 23.76 per 100,000 person-years (UK)	Meniscal tears are very common injuries of the knee The rubbery fibrocartilaginous meniscus, with a cushioning role in the knee, is ruptured The highest incidence is in athletes participating in contact sports Normally results from strong, rapid twisting or hyperflexion of the knee joint Characterised by strong pain, inflammation and tenderness in the knee area May occur with a popping sound
Patellar tendinopathy (jumper's knee)	0.88 per 10,000 athlete exposures (US) 0.12 injuries per 1000 hours among elite athletes (EU)	This is a painful injury associated with overuse of the patellar tendon Pain is activity related and is often located below the patella in the proximal region of the tendon Occurs most frequently in jumping athletes Short-term overuse may result in a reactive tendon that normalises with load adjustment, but high load may lead to chronic injury

Common injuries	Incidence	Characteristics
Ankle sprain	215 per 100,000 person-years (US) 52.7–60.9 per 10,000 person-years (UK)	Reported as the most common ankle injury The ankle ligaments are stretched beyond their limits and in some cases may rupture Athletes who frequently participate in running and jumping sports are at the highest risk for ankle sprains The injury may be short-term with complete recovery, or it may result in long-term disability
Plantar fasciitis	10.5 per 1000 person-years (US)	This degenerative disease of the plantar fascia results in stabbing pain at the heel and plantar side of the foot It is estimated to affect a tenth of the population at some point in their lifetime, with the most commonly affected demographic being middle-aged people Inconsistent leg length, nerve entrapment, muscle tightness, excessive pronation, over-training and uncomfortable footwear are recognised risk factors for plantar fasciitis
Peroneal tendinitis	35% of asymptomatic cases	An injury, resulting from ankle overuse, with pain at the lateral portion The peroneal tendons are inflamed Frequently affects athletes involved in sports with repetitive ankle motion excessive, eversion and pronation

Sources: Bollen (2000); Bridgman (2003); Pedowitz et al. (2003); Clayton and Court-Brown (2008); Scher et al. (2009); Waterman et al. (2010); Swenson et al. (2013); Reinking (2016); Sanders et al. (2016); Bliss (2017); Davda et al. (2017); De Vries et al. (2017); Gans et al. (2018); Khan et al. (2018); Raj and Bubnis (2018); Santana et al. (2018)

Red flags

It is good practice for therapists to familiarise themselves with the red flags for serious pathology in the lower extremity before pursuing manipulative interventions (WHO, 2005). Red flag symptoms help practitioners to identify potentially serious pathology early and exercise sound clinical judgement to avert any potential harm to the patient. Whenever a combination of the red flags in Table 1.6 is observed, manual therapists should refer patients for further clinical screening.

Table 1.6 Red flags for serious pathology in the knee, ankle and foot

Condition	Signs and symptoms
Knee fracture	History of recent trauma to the knee
	Intense localised swelling with effusion and ecchymosis
	Severe tenderness along the joint line
	Flexion less than 90°
	Patient unable to walk more than four weight-bearing steps
Compartment syndrome	History of blunt trauma
	Cumulative trauma
	Overuse
	Intense, persistent pain and firmness to anterior shin compartment
	Reduced pulse
	Paraesthesia
	Pain with toe dorsiflexion
	Intense pain associated with stretch on affected muscles
Extensor mechanism disruption	Quadriceps or patella tendon rupture
	Superior translation of the patella
Fractures	Trauma from a motor vehicle accident, blunt force to the ankle or a fall
	Inflammation on affected leg with concomitant pain
	Relentless synovitis
	Involved tissues feel sore and are highly sensitive
	Difficulty walking more than four weight-bearing steps
Deep vein thrombosis	Recent surgery, period of limited mobility, pregnancy or malignancy
	Hot, erythemic and very tender calf
	Fever and malaise
	Positive Homans sign
	Pain exaggerated with use of the extremity (i.e. walking or standing) and diminished with rest
Septic arthritis	Fever and chills accompanied by consistent pain
	History of bacterial infection
	Recent invasive medical intervention (e.g. surgery or injection)
	Open wound
	Joint inflammation with no history of trauma
	General malaise or loss of appetite
	Compromised immunity
Cancer	Chronic pain with no history of trauma
	History of malignancy
	Weight loss with no clear explanation
	General malaise with or without fever and weakness
	Presence of swelling or unexplained presence of tumours and deformity

Sources: Boissonnault (2005); Stephenson (2013); Magee (2014); Wise (2015)

Special tests

Table 1.7 Special tests for knee, ankle and foot dysfunction

Test	Procedure	Positive sign	Interpretation	Test statistics
Lachman/ Trillat/ Ritchie test	In this one-plane test, the patient assumes a supine posture. The patient's foot is stabilised between the therapist's thigh and the couch. With the therapist's outside hand stabilising the femur, he/she applies gentle force pulling the tibia forward, with the intent of generating anterior translation.	Excessive anterior excursion of the tibia on the femur accompanied by a soft or absent joint end-feel. Diminishing of the normal slope of the infrapatellar tendon	Anterior cruciate ligament injury May also indicate injury to the posterior oblique ligament or arcuate-popliteus complex	Specificity: 0.91 Sensitivity: 0.86
Posterior drawer test	With the patient lying supine, the hip and knee are flexed at 45° and 90° respectively with the tibia in neutral rotation. The therapist pushes backwards on the tibia after stabilising the patient's foot.	Posterior movement of the tibia relative to the femur	Posterior cruciate ligament laxity	Specificity: 0.99 Sensitivity: 0.90
Abduction/ Valgus stress test	In this one-plane medial instability assessment, the therapist pushes the patient's knee medially (valgus stress) while stabilising the ankle in slight lateral rotation. The knee is typically in full extension and 30° flexion. The test thigh may be rested on the table to help the patient relax.	Medial collateral ligament laxity on application of valgus stress	Injury to posterior and medial cruciate ligaments	Specificity: not reported Sensitivity: 0.91

McMurray's test	The patient assumes a supine position with the knee in full flexion. The therapist rotates the tibia medially while extending the knee. The therapist repeatedly changes the amount of flexion while applying medial rotation and then extension to the tibia to test the complete posterior aspect of the meniscus (i.e. posterior horn to middle segment).	A snap or click accompanied by pain	Loose meniscal fragment	Specificity: 0.93 Sensitivity: 0.59
Talar tilt test	The patient lies supine or on the side with the foot relaxed. The normal side is tested first to establish a point of comparison. With the therapist holding the foot at 90°, the talus is tilted from side to side into inversion and eversion.	An increased talar tilt or joint laxity when compared with the normal side	Torn calcaneofibular ligament	Specificity: 0.74 Sensitivity: 0.52
Thompson's/ Simmonds' test	The patient assumes a prone position or kneels on a chair with the feet hanging over the edge of the chair. With the patient relaxed, the therapist squeezes the calf muscles.	Absence of plantarflexion when the calf muscle is squeezed	Achilles tendon rupture	Specificity: 0.93 Sensitivity: 0.96

Test	Procedure	Positive sign	Interpretation	Test statistics
Anterior drawer test	With the patient lying prone, the ankle in a neutral position and the foot in 20° of plantarflexion, the therapist applies an anteriorly directed force to the calcaneus. This may also be done by pushing backwards on the tibia.	Increased anterior translation compared to the normal side	Anterior talocrural joint laxity	Specificity: 0.38 Sensitivity: 0.74
Kleiger test (external rotation stress test)	The patient is seated while flexing the knee at 90°. The therapist stabilises the leg with one hand and applies a passive lateral rotational stress externally to the affected foot and ankle.	Significant pain at the anterolateral part of the distal tibiofibular syndesmosis	Syndesmotic injury Deltoid ligament injury	Specificity: 0.85 Sensitivity: 0.20

Sources: Malanga et al. (2003); Hoskins et al. (2006); Ostrowski (2006); Hattam and Smeatham (2010); de César et al. (2011); Croy et al. (2013); Douglas et al. (2013); Schwieterman et al. (2013); Slaughter et al. (2014)

References

Blackwood, C.B., Yuen, T.J., Sangeorzan, B.J. and Ledoux, W.R. (2005) The midtarsal joint locking mechanism. *Foot and Ankle International 26*, 12, 1074–1080. https://doi.org/10.1177/107110070502601213

Bliss, J.P. (2017) Anterior cruciate ligament injury, reconstruction, and the optimization of outcome. *Indian Journal of Orthopaedics 51*, 606–613. https://doi.org/10.4103/ortho.IJOrtho_237_17

Boissonnault, W.G. (2005) *Primary Care for the Physical Therapist.* Elsevier Saunders.

Bollen, S. (2000) Epidemiology of knee injuries: Diagnosis and triage. *British Journal of Sports Medicine 34*, 227–228.

Bonnel, F., Bonnin, M., Canovas, F., Chamoun, M. and Bouysset, M. (1998) Anatomy of the Foot and Ankle. In M. Bouysset (ed.) *Bone and Joint Disorders of the Foot and Ankle: A Rheumatological Approach.* Springer.

Bridgman, S.A. (2003) Population based epidemiology of ankle sprains attending accident and emergency units in the West Midlands of England, and a survey of UK practice for severe ankle sprains. *Emergency Medicine Journal 20*, 6, 508–510. https://doi.org/10.1136/emj.20.6.508

Brockett, C.L. and Chapman, G.J. (2016) Biomechanics of the ankle. *Orthopaedics and Trauma* 30, 3, 232–238.

Card, R.K. and Bordoni, B. (2019) Anatomy, Bony Pelvis and Lower Limb, Foot Muscles. Stat-Pearls [Internet], www.ncbi.nlm.nih.gov/books/NBK539705

Clanton, T.O. and Paul, P. (2002) Syndesmosis injuries in athletes. *Foot and Ankle Clinics* 7, 3, 529–549.

Clayton, R.A.E. and Court-Brown, C.M. (2008) The epidemiology of musculoskeletal tendinous and ligamentous injuries. *Injury* 39, 1338–1344. https://doi.org/10.1016/j.injury.2008.06.021

Croy, T., Koppenhaver, S., Saliba, S. and Hertel, J. (2013) Anterior talocrural joint laxity: Diagnostic accuracy of the anterior drawer test of the ankle. *Journal of Orthopaedic and Sports Physical Therapy* 43, 12, 911–919. https://doi.org/10.2519/jospt.2013.4679

Davda, K., Malhotra, K., O'Donnell, P., Singh, D. and Cullen, N. (2017) Peroneal tendon disorders. *EFORT Open Reviews* 2, 6, 281–292. https://doi.org/10.1302/2058-5241.2.160047

de César, P.C., Ávila, E.M. and de Abreu, M.R. (2011) Comparison of magnetic resonance imaging to physical examination for syndesmotic injury after lateral ankle sprain. *Foot and Ankle International* 32, 12, 1110–1114. https://doi.org/10.3113/FAI.2011.1110

De Vries, A.J., Koolhaas, W., Zwerver, J., Diercks, R.L. *et al.* (2017) The impact of patellar tendinopathy on sports and work performance in active athletes. *Research in Sports Medicine* 25, 3, 253–265. https://doi.org/10.1080/15438627.2017.1314292

Douglas, G., Nicol, F. and Robertson, C. (eds) (2013) *Macleod's Clinical Examination*, 13th edn. Churchill Livingstone Elsevier.

Ferguson, R., Culliford, D., Prieto-Alhambra, D., Pinedo-Villanueva, R. *et al.* (2019) Encounters for foot and ankle pain in UK primary care: A population-based cohort study of CPRD data. *British Journal of General Practice* 69, 683, e422–e429.

Ficke, J. and Byerly, D.W. (2020) Anatomy, Bony Pelvis and Lower Limb, Foot. StatPearls [Internet], www.ncbi.nlm.nih.gov/books/NBK546698

Gans, I., Retzky, J.S., Jones, L.C. and Tanaka, M.J. (2018) Epidemiology of recurrent anterior cruciate ligament injuries in National Collegiate Athletic Association sports: The Injury Surveillance Program, 2004–2014. *Orthopaedic Journal of Sports Medicine* 6, 232596711877782. https://doi.org/10.1177/2325967118777823

Giangarra, C.E. and Manske, R.C. (eds) (2018) *Clinical Orthopaedic Rehabilitation: A Team Approach*, 4th edn. Elsevier.

Golanó, P., Vega, J., De Leeuw, P.A., Malagelada, F. *et al.* (2010) Anatomy of the ankle ligaments: A pictorial essay. *Knee Surgery, Sports Traumatology, Arthroscopy* 18, 5, 557–569.

Hattam, P. and Smeatham, A. (2010) *Special Tests in Musculoskeletal Examination: An Evidence-Based Guide for Clinicians*. Churchill Livingstone Elsevier.

Hoskins, W., McHardy, A., Pollard, H., Windsham, R. and Onley, R. (2006) Chiropractic treatment of lower extremity conditions: A literature review. *Journal of Manipulative Physiological Therapeutics* 29, 8, 658–671. https://doi.org/10.1016/j.jmpt.2006.08.004

Khan, I.A. and Varacallo, M. (2019) Anatomy, Bony Pelvis and Lower Limb, Foot Talus. StatPearls [Internet], www.ncbi.nlm.nih.gov/books/NBK541086

Khan, T., Alvand, A., Prieto-Alhambra, D., Culliford, D.J. *et al.* (2018) ACL and meniscal injuries increase the risk of primary total knee replacement for osteoarthritis: A matched case-control study using the Clinical Practice Research Datalink (CPRD). *British Journal of Sports Medicine* 53, 15, 1–5. https://doi.org/10.1136/bjsports-2017-097762

Krähenbühl, N., Horn-Lang, T., Hintermann, B. and Knupp, M. (2017) The subtalar joint: A complex mechanism. *EFORT Open Reviews* 2, 7, 309–316.

Magee, D.J. (2014) *Orthopedic Physical Assessment*, 6th edn. Saunders.

Magee, D.J., Zachazewski, J.E., Quillen, W.S. and Manske, R.C. (2016) *Pathology and Intervention in Musculoskeletal Rehabilitation, Pathology and Intervention in Musculoskeletal Rehabilitation*, 2nd edn. Elsevier. https://doi.org/10.1016/c2012-0-05970-4

Malanga, G.A., Andrus, S., Nadler, S.F. and McLean, J. (2003) Physical examination of the knee: A review of the original test description and scientific validity of common orthopedic tests. *Archives of Physical Medicine and Rehabilitation 84*, 592–603.

Manganaro, D., Dollinger, B., Nezwek, T.A. and Sadiq, N.M. (2019) Anatomy, Bony Pelvis and Lower Limb, Foot Joints. StatPearls [Internet], www.ncbi.nlm.nih.gov/books/NBK536941

Moore, K.L., Dalley, A.F. and Agur, A.M. (2013) Lower Limb. In *Clinically Oriented Anatomy*, 7th edn. Lippincott Williams & Wilkins.

Mróz, I., Kurzydło, W., Bachul, P., Jaworek, J. *et al.* (2015) Inferior tibiofibular joint (tibiofibular syndesmosis) – own studies and review of the literature. *Folia Medica Cracoviensia 55*, 4, 71–79.

Norkin, C.C. and White, D.J. (2009) *Measurement of Joint Motion: A Guide to Goniometry*. F.A. Davis.

Oatis, C.A. (1988) Biomechanics of the foot and ankle under static conditions. *Physical Therapy 68*, 12, 1815–1821.

Ostrowski, J.A. (2006) Accuracy of 3 diagnostic tests for anterior cruciate ligament tears. *Journal of Athletic Training 41*, 1, 120–121.

Pedowitz, R.A., O'Connor, J.J. and Akeson, W.H. (eds) (2003) *Daniel's Knee Injuries: Ligament and Cartilage Structure, Function, Injury, and Repair*, 2nd edn. Lippincott Williams & Wilkins.

Raj, M.A. and Bubnis, M.A. (2018) Knee Meniscal Tears. StatPearls [Internet], www.ncbi.nlm.nih.gov/books/NBK431067

Reinking, M.F. (2016) Current concepts in the treatment of patellar tendinopathy. *International Journal of Sports Physical Therapy 11*, 6, 854–866.

Sanders, T.L., Maradit Kremers, H., Bryan, A.J., Larson, D.R. *et al.* (2016) Incidence of anterior cruciate ligament tears and reconstruction. *American Journal of Sports Medicine 44*, 6, 1502–1507. https://doi.org/10.1177/0363546516629944

Santana, J.A., Mabrouk, A. and Sherman, A.I. (2018) Jumpers Knee. StatPearls [Internet], https://pubmed.ncbi.nlm.nih.gov/30422564

Scher, C.D.L., Belmont, L.C.P.J., Bear, M.R., Mountcastle, S.B., Orr, J.D. and Owens, M.B.D. (2009) The incidence of plantar fasciitis in the United States military. *Journal of Bone and Joint Surgery 91*, 12, 2867–2872. https://doi.org/10.2106/JBJS.I.00257

Schwieterman, B., Haas, D., Columber, K., Knupp, D. and Cook, C. (2013) Diagnostic accuracy of physical examination tests of the ankle/foot complex: A systematic review. *International Journal of Sports Physical Therapy 8*, 4, 416–426.

Slaughter, A.J., Reynolds, K.A., Jambhekar, K., David, R.M., Hasan, S.A. and Pandey, T. (2014) Clinical orthopedic examination findings in the lower extremity: Correlation with imaging studies and diagnostic efficacy. *RadioGraphics 34*, 2, e41–e55. https://doi.org/10.1148/rg.342125066

Standring, S. (2008) *Gray's Anatomy: The Anatomical Basis of Clinical Practice*, 40th edn. Churchill Livingstone Elsevier.

Standring, S. (2016) *Gray's Anatomy: The Anatomical Basis of Clinical Practice*, 41st edn. Elsevier.

Stephenson, C. (2013) *The Complementary Therapist's Guide to Red Flags and Referrals*. Churchill Livingstone Elsevier.

Swenson, D.M., Collins, C.L., Best, T.M., Flanigan, D.C. *et al.* (2013) Epidemiology of knee injuries among US high school athletes, 2005/2006–2010/2011. *Medicine and Science in Sports and Exercise 45*, 3, 462–469. https://doi.org/10.1249/MSS.0b013e318277acca

Tang, A. and Bordoni, B. (2021) Anatomy, Bony Pelvis and Lower Limb, Foot Nerves. StatPearls [Internet], www.ncbi.nlm.nih.gov/books/NBK537292

Tate, P. (2009) Anatomy of Bones and Joints. In *Seeley's Principles of Anatomy and Physiology*. McGraw-Hill.

Thomas, M.J., Roddy, E., Zhang, W., Menz, H.B., Hannan, M.T. and Peat, G.M. (2011) The population prevalence of foot and ankle pain in middle and old age: A systematic review. *Pain 152*, 12, 2870–2880.

Tweed, J.L., Campbell, J.A., Thompson, R.J. and Curran, M.J. (2008) The function of the mid-tarsal joint: A review of the literature. *The Foot* 18, 2, 106–112.

Waterman, C.B.R., Owens, M.B.D., Davey, C.S., Zacchilli, C.M.A. and Belmont, L.C.P.J. (2010) The epidemiology of ankle sprains in the United States. *Journal of Bone and Joint Surgery* 92, 13, 2279–2284. https://doi.org/10.2106/JBJS.I.01537

Wise, C.H. (2015) *Orthopaedic Manual Physical Therapy: From Art to Evidence*. F.A. Davis Company.

World Health Organization (WHO) (2005) *WHO Guidelines on Basic Training and Safety in Chiropractic*. WHO, www.wfc.org/website/index.php?option=com_content&view=article&id=110&lang=en

Young, R., Nix, S., Wholohan, A., Bradhurst, R. and Reed, L. (2013) Interventions for increasing ankle joint dorsiflexion: A systematic review and meta-analysis. *Journal of Foot and Ankle Research* 6, 46. https://doi.org/10.1186/1757-1146-6-46

Chapter 2

Biomechanics of the Foot and Ankle

The ankle and foot, owing to their location, form the kinetic linkage that allows the lower extremity to interact with the ground. This dynamic link between the body and the earth is a basic requirement for all our upright locomotion and other activities of daily living. The ankle and foot complex adapts to uneven surfaces, working synchronously with other structures of the lower limb, and constantly withstands high compressive and shear forces during different phases of the gait cycle. The bony, muscular and ligamentous structures of this complex provide leverage for propulsion and traction for movement with a high degree of stability. Proper movement within this complex also decreases the forces of weight-bearing during gait with dorsiflexion (Donatelli, 1985; Rodgers, 1988; Chan and Rudins, 1994).

The ankle and foot complex, however, is highly susceptible to pain, trauma/stress and other injuries. These injuries can cause long-term disability and are a potential source of morbidity in both general people and elite athletes. In the United States, every year injuries to this complex account for over 3 million emergency department visits (Cherry *et al.*, 2009; Reissig *et al.*, 2017). In the United Kingdom, the prevalence of foot and ankle pain across all age groups is about 3% (2980 per 100,000); of these, the most commonly affected patient groups were women (54.4%) and the older population (71–80 years) (Ferguson *et al.*, 2019). In fact, in the elderly population, foot and ankle problems affect about one in every four people and significantly impact the ability to do activities of daily living and health-related quality of life (Benvenuti *et al.*, 1995; Mickle *et al.*, 2011; Thomas *et al.*, 2011; Menz, 2015). In addition, according to the UK Clinical Practice Research Datalink, ankle and foot pain accounts for, on average, 8500 referrals to physiotherapists annually (Ferguson *et al.*, 2019).

Most problems in the ankle and foot complex have a chronic component to their origin. In general, inadequate distribution of various forces (e.g. compressive, tensile, shearing and rotatory forces) generated during the gait cycle places undue stress on this complex, which eventually causes the gradual wear and tear of connective tissue and muscle. The repetitive forces absorbed by this complex may over time lead to stress fracture, localised cartilage breakdown, joint instability, tendinitis and ligamentous laxity (Donatelli, 1985; Chan and Rudins, 1994; Towers *et al.*, 2003). This is analogous to a rope that breaks over time if it is repetitively pulled in an eccentric manner. Hence, to avoid misdiagnosis and ensure correct treatment of this complex, it is essential to understand the amount and type of forces the ankle and foot normally subject themselves to given their variations in weight, type and activities from person to person. This chapter therefore discusses the basic biomechanics and normal alignment of the ankle and foot complex that are relevant to manual therapists.

Motion of the ankle and foot

The motion of the ankle and foot complex is multiplanar and broadly includes three cardinal planes: sagittal, transverse and frontal planes. Motions within the sagittal plane, about the X-axis, are plantarflexion (downward) and dorsiflexion (upward). Abduction (valgus) and adduction (varus) are the movements in the transverse or axial plane, about the cephalocaudal Y-axis. Motions that occur in the frontal or coronal plane, about the anteroposterior Z-axis, are eversion and inversion (Towers *et al.*, 2003). The components of these three motions, however, do not function in isolation as individual movements; in fact, they act simultaneously as a unit in a synchronised and coordinated manner. Thus, all motion within the ankle and foot complex is essentially triplane motion (Chan and Rudins, 1994; Nordin and Frankel, 2001).

The combinations of these motions create three-dimensional motions, which are termed in the literature as supination and pronation. Both terms also describe the position of the sole. The term 'supination of the foot' refers to the combined movement of adduction, plantarflexion and inversion. This combination causes the sole to face medially. In contrast, the 'pronation of the foot' includes abduction, dorsiflexion and eversion movements, which position the sole to face laterally. Supination and pronation are commonly described as an open kinetic chain. These movements occur at certain points during the stance phase of the gait cycle. They primarily help reduce the forces of weight-bearing and stabilise numerous joints within the lower extremity. There are five triplanar joints within the ankle and foot complex that permit supination and pronation: the subtalar joint, the midtarsal joint, the tibiotalar joint, the first metatarsal joint and the fifth metatarsal joint (Donatelli, 1985; Towers *et al.*, 2003; Brockett and Chapman, 2016).

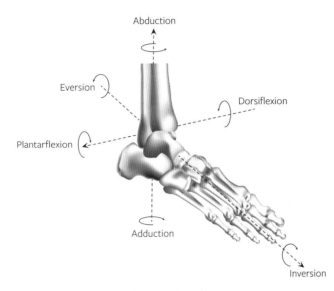

Figure 2.1 Foot and ankle movements

Range of motion

The range of motion (ROM) at the ankle varies greatly between individuals owing to cultural and geographical differences, which have a direct influence on the activities of daily living (Kumar *et al.*, 2011). Most of the ankle movements occur primarily in the sagittal plane, providing the majority of plantarflexion and dorsiflexion. The axis of rotation of the ankle is dynamic due to the complex morphology of the talocrural joint, which permits substantial internal rotation in coordination with the subtalar joint (Towers *et al.*, 2003). Hence, the ankle also allows some degrees of motion at the frontal plane (see Table 2.1). The motion of the subtalar joint is triplanar, providing pronation and supination. The joint allows 1° of freedom.

In our activities of daily living, however, considerably less ROM from the above data is required in the sagittal plane (walking: maximum 30°; ascending and descending stairs: about 37° and 56°, respectively) (Nordin and Frankel, 2001).

The range of motion of the foot is complex. The midtarsal joints (or

Chopart's joints) allow some degrees of inversion and eversion but mainly serve to amplify the motions of the talocrural joint and the subtalar joint (Oatis, 1988). The motion of the tarsometatarsal joints is translatory or planar. The metatarsophalangeal joints have about 2° of freedom, allowing motion in the sagittal and transverse planes. The interphalangeal joints permit motion in the sagittal plane, allowing pure flexion and extension (Norkin and White, 2009).

Table 2.1 Ankle range of motion

Plane type	ROM (in degrees)	Movements	Range (in degrees)	References
Sagittal plane	65–75 (overall)	Dorsiflexion	10–20	Grimston *et al.* (1993)
		Plantarflexion	40–55	
Frontal plane	35 (approximately)	Inversion	23	Stauffer *et al.* (1977); Brockett and Chapman (2016)
		Eversion	12	

Table 2.2 Range of motion of the foot

Joint name	Movement type	Range of motion (in degrees)
Subtalar joint	Inversion	0–50
	Eversion	0–26
Metatarsophalangeal joints	Flexion (hallux)	0–45
	Extension (hallux)	0–80
	Flexion (lesser toes)	0–40
	Extension (lesser toes)	0–70
Interphalangeal joints	Flexion (hallux)	0–90
	Flexion (lesser toes)	0–30
	Extension (hallux and other toes)	0–80

Sources: Oatis (1988); Norkin and White (2009)

Foot and ankle kinematics during gait

The ankle and foot complex has special qualities to be rigid and flexible as needed. It becomes flexible to absorb load when the foot is in contact with the ground. This allows it to move with more freedom and adapt to uneven surfaces. The foot becomes rigid like a lever arm when it is about to leave the ground. This enables the lower limb to propel forward with body weight (Towers *et al.*, 2003; Van Hulle *et al.*, 2020). These tasks of flexibility and rigidity are the main highlights of the gait cycle, which is briefly reviewed here.

The gait cycle is the time interval between two footsteps (i.e. the time interval between the two successive first ground contacts or heel strikes of the same foot). The walking cycle of gait can be broadly divided into two phases.

The stance phase is the entire period in which the foot is on the ground. It represents about 60–62% of the total gait cycle and serves to permit weight-bearing and ensure limb stability. This phase begins when the foot first makes contact with the ground and ends with the ipsilateral foot leaving the ground. The stance phase takes approximately 0.59–0.67 seconds during an average walking cycle (Alamdari and Krovi, 2017). In addition, unlike the running cycle, both feet stay on the ground at the same time for a brief period (about 10%) of the walking stance phase. This phase includes five distinct stages: heel-strike (HS), foot-flat (FF), mid-stance (MS), heel-off (HO) or push-off, and toe-off (TO) (Rodgers, 1988). Functionally, it includes four intervals: initial contact, loading response, mid-stance and terminal stance (Silva and Stergiou, 2020).

The swing phase is the period in which the same foot becomes non-weight-bearing as it is in the air. This phase starts as soon as the foot is lifted off the ground and ends when the ipsilateral foot touches the ground. It constitutes about 38–40% of the total gait cycle and allows the forward momentum for the lower limb (Alamdari and Krovi, 2017). It also makes the foot ready for heel strike with proper alignment to ensure the swinging foot clears the floor. This phase takes, on average, 0.38–0.42 seconds during the walking cycle and has four functional intervals: pre-swing, initial swing, mid-swing and terminal swing (Kawalec, 2017; Laribi and Zeghloul, 2020).

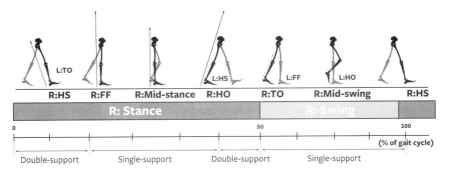

Figure 2.2 Stance and swing phases of the walking cycle

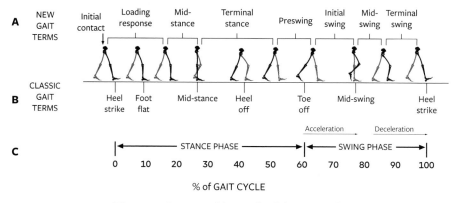

Figure 2.3 Stages and intervals of the gait cycle

Table 2.3 Different stages/intervals of the stance and swing phases during the gait cycle

Stages/intervals	Characteristics
Heel-strike (or initial contact)	Start: the moment the heel makes the initial contact with the ground
	End: until the whole foot touches the ground
	Represents 0–2% of the gait cycle
	First instance of double-leg support
	Lower-limb motion: internal rotation of the lower limb; 30° flexion of the hip; 5° medial rotation of the tibia; full extension of the knee; and neutral position (supinated 5°) or slight plantarflexion of the ankle
Foot-flat (or loading response)	Start: when the whole foot touches the ground
	End: when the centre of gravity is directly over the top foot
	Represents 2–12% of the gait cycle
	Performs the task of weight acceptance by allowing the foot to cushion the force of weight-bearing
	Lower-limb motion: the lower limb begins rotating laterally with gradual extension of the hip, 15–20° knee flexion and 10–15° ankle plantarflexion
Mid-stance	Start: when centre of gravity is directly over the ankle joint
	End: the moment the heel starts to lift off the surface
	Represents 12–31% of the gait cycle
	First part of the body's single-leg support period
	Transforms the foot into a rigid lever to propel the body forward
	Lower-limb motion: the lower limb reverses into external rotation; the heel inverts; the hip moves from flexion to extension; maximal flexion of the knee; and supination and dorsiflexion (5°) of the ankle

Heel-off (or terminal stance)	Start: when the heel begins to leave the ground End: when the contralateral foot touches the ground Represents 31–50% of the gait cycle Second part of the body's single-leg support period Prepares the foot for the forward propulsion of the body Transforms the force of weight-bearing into kinetic energy Lower-limb motion: maximal external rotation of the lower limb; the heel inverts maximally; maximum intrinsic muscle and plantar flexor activity; 10–13° of hip hyperextension; around 0–5° of knee flexion; and supination and plantarflexion of the ankle
Toe-off (or pre-swing)	Start: the moment the toes begin to lift off the ground End: when the toes leave the ground and are in the air Represents 50–60% of the gait cycle End of the stance phase and start of the swing phase Second instance of loading period and double-leg support Lower-limb motion: the lower limb starts rotating medially with less hip extension; 35–40° flexion of the knee; 20° plantarflexion of the ankle; the eversion of heel; and unlocking of the transverse tarsal joint
Initial swing	Start: when toes are off the ground End: when the knee flexes maximally Represents 60–73% of the gait cycle First part of the swing period Prepares the limb for forward advancement Lower-limb motion: the lower limb rotates medially; 10° hip extension and then 20° flexion due to contraction of the iliopsoas muscle; 40–60° knee flexion; ankle dorsiflexes and then ends in a neutral position
Mid-swing	Start: the moment the knee flexes maximally End: until the tibia is vertical to the surface Represents 74–87% of the gait cycle Second part of the swing period Continues the limb advancement Makes the foot ready for next ground contact Enables the foot to clear the ground Lower-limb motion: the lower limb continues to rotate medially; 30° flexion of the hip; dorsiflexion of the ankle; 60° flexion initially but then around 30° extension of the knee
Terminal swing	Start: the moment the tibia gets vertical to the ground End: when the foot makes the next ground contact with heel strike Represents 85–100% of the gait cycle Final part of the swing period Makes the final advancement of the limb Positions the foot for initial contact Lower-limb motion: the lower limb continues rotating medially; 25–30° hip flexion; locked knee extension; and neutral ankle position

Sources: Rodgers (1988); Loudon et al. (2008); Perry and Burnfield (2010); Shultz et al. (2015); Alamdari and Krovi (2017); Silva and Stergiou (2020)

Abnormal gait: effects on hip, knee and ankle

Abnormal gait patterns are walking abnormalities that may occur for many reasons, including muscle weakness, altered joint load, degenerative processes, anatomic deformities, injuries or other impairments. Many factors, however, play a role that may lead to gait abnormalities. Three of the key factors influencing a person's gait pattern include age, personality and mood (Mielke *et al.*, 2013; Pirker and Katzenschlager, 2017). The prevalence of gait disorders greatly increases with age, as elderly people are more likely to have slower motor reactions, weaker muscles and poorer lower-limb coordination compared to younger people (Verghese *et al.*, 2014). Studying a large cohort of community-residing elderly, Mahlknecht *et al.* (2013) suggested that in the older population, gait abnormalities increase from 10% in the 60s to more than 60% in the 80s. Table 2.4 lists some of the common gait abnormalities.

Table 2.4 Common abnormalities of gait

Abnormal gait patterns	Characteristics	Aetiology
Antalgic gait	The most common type of gait abnormality A shortened stance phase but lengthened swing phase on the injured side Causes the affected patient to limp due to pain in weight-bearing structures of the affected leg The foot lifts off and contacts the ground in a fixed ankle position Likely impairments: knee joint contractures, hip extensor weakness, hip flexor contractures, plantar flexor contracture or ankle dorsiflexor weakness (Perry and Burnfield, 2010; Colgan *et al.*, 2016)	Often results from painful conditions of the lower back or the lower limb (e.g. knee or hip osteoarthritis, spinal osteomyelitis, stress fractures, ankle sprains) (Auerbach and Tadi, 2021)
Ataxic gait (cerebellar)	Clumsy, wobbly or uncoordinated walk with a wide-based gait The foot may fall forwards, backwards or side to side Inability to walk in a straight line Mostly resembles the gait of acute alcohol intoxication About 10,000 adults and 500 children are affected by this gait in the UK (Wardle and Robertson, 2007; Musselman *et al.*, 2014) The Romberg's sign will be positive Limb ataxia often defines hemisphere lesions while trunk instability indicates midline cerebellar disease involving vermis lesions Pathomechanism: balance and motor control disturbances (Buckley *et al.*, 2018; Zhang *et al.*, 2021)	Has an association with cerebellar disturbances Causes may include long-term alcohol abuse, degenerative disease, vascular condition, neoplasm, etc. (Pirker and Katzenschlager, 2017)

Ataxic gait (sensory)	Loss of proprioception (i.e. ability to perceive movement and location)	Impairment of somatosensory nerve
	Eyes often compensate for the lack of proprioception in these patients	Any abnormalities affecting the afferent pathway between the peripheral nerve and the parietal cortex
	High steps, shortened step length and hard feet slapping	
	Gait is sluggish, broad-based, more cautious and insecure	Disorders of the dorsal columns (e.g. cobalamin deficiency) (Zhang *et al.*, 2021)
	May have a stomping quality as the legs are lifted high	
	The severe form resembles the cerebellar ataxic gait (Pirker and Katzenschlager, 2017; Ramdharry, 2018)	
Waddling gait	A waddling, duck-like walk due to exaggerated movement of the trunk and excessive elevation of the hip	Hip disorders (e.g. hip dysplasia, bilateral Perthes, septic sequelae)
	The pelvis drops from its level while walking (Trendelenburg sign)	Pelvic girdle and upper thigh muscle weakness
	Difficulty in standing up from a sitting position	Muscular dystrophy
	May also occur in patients with myopathies (Lim *et al.*, 2007; Suresh and Wimalaratna, 2013)	Presence of hip dislocation from birth (Sharma *et al.*, 2020)
Equine gait (steppage gait)	The leg is lifted higher than normal and the foot drops while walking	Often results from peroneal neuropathies (e.g. peroneal nerve palsy, lumbosacral radiculopathy, peroneal muscle atrophy), cerebral vascular accident or amyotrophic lateral sclerosis (Nori and Das, 2020)
	The toes point downward during the swing phase and scrape the ground while making the initial contact	
	Loss of foot dorsiflexion	
	The affected patient walks mostly by flexing the hip joint	
	Inability to stand or walk on the heel (Bowley and Doughty, 2018)	
Diplegic gait (spastic gait)	Walking with an abnormally narrow base, a 'scissor'-type gait	Underlying cause is unknown
	Primarily affects both legs with equinus deformity of the foot	Associated with congenital brain malformations, blood problems to the brain, genetic abnormalities, etc. (Rana *et al.*, 2017)
	The legs are very stiff, dragged in a semicircular motion, and the toes scrape the ground	
	Lack of stability in standing and walking	
	Loss of plantarflexion in loading response and pre-swing and dorsiflexion in mid-stance	
	Common in those with cerebral palsy or multiple sclerosis (Whittle, 2007; Gage *et al.*, 2009)	
	Likely impairments: contractures of the adductor muscles; overactivity of the hamstrings, triceps surae and triceps peronei (Whittle, 2007)	

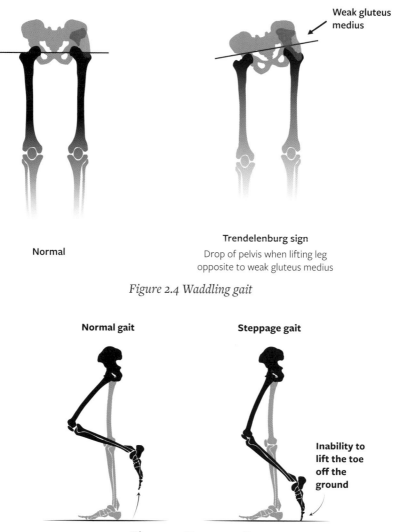

Figure 2.4 *Waddling gait*

Figure 2.5 *Steppage gait*

References

Alamdari, A. and Krovi, V.N. (2017) A Review of Computational Musculoskeletal Analysis of Human Lower Extremities. In J. Ueda and Y. Kurita (eds) *Human Modelling for Bio-Inspired Robotics*. Elsevier.

Auerbach, N. and Tadi, P. (2021) Antalgic Gait in Adults. StatPearls [Internet], www.ncbi.nlm.nih.gov/books/NBK559243

Benvenuti, F., Ferrucci, L., Guralnik, J.M., Gangemi, S. and Baroni, A. (1995) Foot pain and disability in older persons: An epidemiologic survey. *Journal of the American Geriatrics Society* 43, 5, 479–484.

Bowley, M.P. and Doughty, C.T. (2018) Entrapment neuropathies of the lower extremity. *The Medical Clinics of North America 103*, 2, 371–382.

Brockett, C.L. and Chapman, G.J. (2016) Biomechanics of the ankle. *Orthopaedics and Trauma 30*, 3, 232–238.

Buckley, E., Mazzà, C. and McNeill, A. (2018) A systematic review of the gait characteristics associated with Cerebellar Ataxia. *Gait and Posture 60*, 154–163.

Chan, C.W. and Rudins, A. (1994) Foot biomechanics during walking and running. *Mayo Clinic Proceedings 69*, 5, 448–461.

Cherry, D.K., Hing, E., Woodwell, D.A. and Rechtsteiner, E.A. (2009) National ambulatory medical care survey: 2006 summary. *National Health Statistics Reports*, No. 3. National Center for Health Statistics.

Colgan, G., Walsh, M., Bennett, D., Rice, J. and O'Brien, T. (2016) Gait analysis and hip extensor function early post total hip replacement. *Journal of Orthopaedics 13*, 3, 171–176.

Donatelli, R. (1985) Normal biomechanics of the foot and ankle. *Journal of Orthopaedic and Sports Physical Therapy 7*, 3, 91–95.

Ferguson, R., Culliford, D., Prieto-Alhambra, D., Pinedo-Villanueva, R. *et al.* (2019) Encounters for foot and ankle pain in UK primary care: A population-based cohort study of CPRD data. *British Journal of General Practice 69*, 683, e422–e429.

Gage, J.R., Schwartz, M.H., Koop, S.E. and Novacheck, T.F. (eds) (2009) *The Identification and Treatment of Gait Problems in Cerebral Palsy*. Mac Keith Press.

Grimston, S.K., Nigg, B.M., Hanley, D.A. and Engsberg, J.R. (1993) Differences in ankle joint complex range of motion as a function of age. *Foot and Ankle 14*, 4, 215–222.

Kawalec, J.S. (2017) Mechanical Testing of Foot and Ankle Implants. In E. Friis (ed.) *Mechanical Testing of Orthopaedic Implants*. Woodhead Publishing.

Kumar, S., Sharma, R., Gulati, D., Dhammi, I.K. and Aggarwal, A.N. (2011) Normal range of motion of hip and ankle in Indian population. *Acta Orthopaedica et Traumatologica Turcica 45*, 6, 421–424.

Laribi, M.A. and Zeghloul, S. (2020) Human Lower Limb Operation Tracking via Motion Capture Systems. In M. Ceccarelli and G. Carbone (eds) *Design and Operation of Human Locomotion Systems*. Academic Press.

Lim, M.R., Huang, R.C., Wu, A., Girardi, F.P. and Cammisa Jr, F.P. (2007) Evaluation of the elderly patient with an abnormal gait. *Journal of the American Academy of Orthopaedic Surgeons 15*, 2, 107–117.

Loudon, J.K., Swift, M. and Bell, S. (2008) *The Clinical Orthopedic Assessment Guide*. Human Kinetics.

Mahlknecht, P., Kiechl, S., Bloem, B.R., Willeit, J. *et al.* (2013) Prevalence and burden of gait disorders in elderly men and women aged 60–97 years: A population-based study. *PLOS ONE 8*, 7, e69627.

Menz, H.B. (2015) Biomechanics of the ageing foot and ankle: A mini-review. *Gerontology 61*, 4, 381–388.

Mickle, K.J., Munro, B.J., Lord, S.R., Menz, H.B. and Steele, J.R. (2011) Cross-sectional analysis of foot function, functional ability, and health-related quality of life in older people with disabling foot pain. *Arthritis Care and Research 63*, 11, 1592–1598.

Mielke, M.M., Roberts, R.O., Savica, R., Cha, R. *et al.* (2013) Assessing the temporal relationship between cognition and gait: Slow gait predicts cognitive decline in the Mayo Clinic Study of Aging. *Journals of Gerontology Series A: Biomedical Sciences and Medical Sciences 68*, 8, 929–937.

Musselman, K.E., Stoyanov, C.T., Marasigan, R., Jenkins, M.E. *et al.* (2014) Prevalence of ataxia in children: A systematic review. *Neurology 82*, 1, 80–89.

Nordin, M. and Frankel, V.H. (eds) (2001) *Basic Biomechanics of the Musculoskeletal System*. Lippincott Williams & Wilkins.

Nori, S.L. and Das, J.M. (2020) Steppage Gait. StatPearls [Internet], www.ncbi.nlm.nih.gov/books/NBK547672

Norkin, C.C. and White, D.J. (2009) *Measurement of Joint Motion: A Guide to Goniometry*. F.A. Davis.

Oatis, C.A. (1988) Biomechanics of the foot and ankle under static conditions. *Physical Therapy* 68, 12, 1815–1821.

Perry, J. and Burnfield, J.M. (2010) *Gait Analysis: Normal and Pathological Function*. Slack Inc.

Pirker, W. and Katzenschlager, R. (2017) Gait disorders in adults and the elderly. *Wiener Klinische Wochenschrift* 129, 3, 81–95.

Ramdharry, G. (2018) Peripheral nerve disease. *Handbook of Clinical Neurology* 159, 403–415.

Rana, M., Upadhyay, J., Rana, A., Durgapal, S. and Jantwal, A. (2017) A systematic review on etiology, epidemiology, and treatment of cerebral palsy. *International Journal of Nutrition, Pharmacology, Neurological Diseases* 7, 4, 76–83.

Reissig, J., Bitterman, A. and Lee, S. (2017) Common foot and ankle injuries: What not to miss and how best to manage. *Journal of Osteopathic Medicine* 117, 2, 98–104.

Rodgers, M.M. (1988) Dynamic biomechanics of the normal foot and ankle during walking and running. *Physical Therapy* 68, 12, 1822–1830.

Sharma, A., Sinha, S., Narang, A., Chouhan, D.K. and Gupta, S. (2020) Waddling gait: A complication of valproate therapy and a thought beyond vitamin D deficiency. *Sultan Qaboos University Medical Journal* 20, 1, e104–e108.

Shultz, S.J., Houglum, P.A. and Perrin, D.H. (2015) *Examination of Musculoskeletal Injuries*, 4th edn. Human Kinetics.

Silva, L.M. and Stergiou, N. (2020) The Basics of Gait Analysis. In N. Stergiou (ed.) *Biomechanics and Gait Analysis*. Academic Press.

Stauffer, R.N., Chao, E.Y. and Brewster, R.C. (1977) Force and motion analysis of the normal, diseased, and prosthetic ankle joint. *Clinical Orthopaedics and Related Research* 1977, 127, 189–196.

Suresh, E. and Wimalaratna, S. (2013) Proximal myopathy: Diagnostic approach and initial management. *Postgraduate Medical Journal* 89, 1054, 470–477.

Thomas, M.J., Roddy, E., Zhang, W., Menz, H.B., Hannan, M.T. and Peat, G.M. (2011) The population prevalence of foot and ankle pain in middle and old age: A systematic review. *Pain* 152, 12, 2870–2880.

Towers, J.D., Deible, C.T. and Golla, S.K. (2003) Foot and ankle biomechanics. *Seminars in Musculoskeletal Radiology* 7, 1, 67–74.

Van Hulle, R., Schwartz, C., Denoël, V., Croisier, J.L., Forthomme, B. and Brüls, O. (2020) A foot/ground contact model for biomechanical inverse dynamics analysis. *Journal of Biomechanics* 100, 109412.

Verghese, J., Annweiler, C., Ayers, E., Barzilai, N. *et al.* (2014) Motoric cognitive risk syndrome: Multicountry prevalence and dementia risk. *Neurology* 83, 8, 718–726.

Wardle, M. and Robertson, N. (2007) Chronic progressive late onset cerebellar ataxia. *Advances in Clinical Neuroscience and Rehabilitation* 7, 2, 6–12.

Whittle, M.W. (2007) Gait Assessment in Cerebral Palsy. In M.W. Whittle (ed.) *Gait Analysis*, 4th edn. Butterworth-Heinemann.

Zhang, Q., Zhou, X., Li, Y., Yang, X. and Abbasi, Q.H. (2021) Clinical recognition of sensory ataxia and cerebellar ataxia. *Frontiers in Human Neuroscience* 15, 639871.

Chapter 3

Clinical Examination and Special Tests for the Foot and Ankle

The foot and ankle complex is made up of an array of bones, joints, ligaments and tendons that must work synergistically for normal walking and running and to perform weight-bearing while standing. An injury to any of these structures places undue stress on other structures of the lower limb and can interfere with a person's ability to do the activities of daily living. In severe cases, such injuries can even lead to a long-term disability. This has been demonstrated in clinical studies, where foot and ankle injuries were identified as a potential source of morbidity in both general people and elite athletes (Reissig *et al.*, 2017; Ferguson *et al.*, 2019).

Professional sportspersons and recreational exercisers are typically more susceptible to foot and ankle injuries as their physically demanding activities often involve tremendous lower-limb loading (Chinn and Hertel, 2010; Luciano and Lara, 2012). The foot and ankle usually carry a heavy burden because of the amount of torque generated through them during strenuous activities such as running or jumping. These two structures also take the brunt of the repetitive trauma, as they bear high compressive forces and are exposed to repeated structural overuse. Sprains, stress fractures, soft-tissue damage and other bony injuries are thus more common in this region of the lower limb (Hartley and Robinson, 1995; Hunt *et al.*, 2017). Hence, a careful examination of the foot and ankle is essential for the correct diagnosis and management of these injuries.

Examination of the foot and ankle can be challenging for manual therapists, as the patient may present with a diverse range of problems including pain, swelling, muscle spasm, anatomic deformity, structural instability, stiffness, sprain, strain and/or abnormal gait (Davies and Blundell, 2011). In addition, the underlying cause(s) of these presenting symptoms can be anything from minor trauma to degenerative conditions and/or systemic diseases such as diabetes, gout, osteoarthritis, infection, obesity, etc. Hence, there is a high likelihood of false-positive errors during the diagnosis. However, if the therapist follows the basic principles of question, look, feel and move with a logical approach and supplements the diagnosis with appropriate special tests, then the entire assessment process can be simple and rewarding (Young *et al.*, 2005; Bhatia and Aziz, 2020). In fact, with this approach, it is highly likely that the therapist would make a sound clinical judgement in the end.

Gathering valuable data by breaking down the diagnosis into the component parts can help to develop a working hypothesis that may further guide the examination. This may even lead to a referral to a physician or a more experienced clinician due to a red flag. This chapter is therefore written to describe the clinical examination of common musculoskeletal complaints and other pathologies of the foot and ankle. We also discuss some of the commonly used special tests to assess the nature and severity of these problems and the characteristics and limitations of these tests in light of the current scientific evidence.

Clinical examination: how to start

Manual therapists should start examining the patient from the moment he/she walks in for consultation. Patients suffering from foot or ankle pathology can have coexisting conditions, so the therapist should first carefully evaluate the patient's chief complaint, conducting a thorough medical history evaluation. A methodical approach (i.e. look, feel and move) should then be adopted for the physical examination of the foot and ankle. This approach needs to be specific to the patient's complaints so that the symptoms can be reproduced. The therapist should then perform the most appropriate special tests to further confirm the initial findings from the patient interview, inspection and palpation. This should be done as part of the treatment scheme so that the therapist can identify the underlying cause(s) of the patient's presenting condition, rule out the red flags and determine a safe and appropriate treatment plan that will increase the possibility of a positive clinical outcome. Figure 3.1 presents a step-by-step flow diagram on clinical examination and the decision-making process.

Patient interview (history)

Taking a detailed medical history is the most important aspect of a patient interview. This is because the narrative provided by the patient often helps to pinpoint the chief complaint and its possible underlying cause(s). Thus, both the therapist and the patient should be comfortable during the interview. To create such an environment, the consultation room needs to be spacious with a height-adjustable examination table or couch and an area to walk in. The therapist should conduct the history taking in a smooth and structured manner so that they can cover all the key points summarised in Box 3.1 (Ohm *et al.*, 2013; Seitz *et al.*, 2019). For new patients or those with an unconfirmed diagnosis, Alazzawi *et al.* (2017) recommended that therapists should not go through earlier reports or notes before seeing the patient. They suggested that, with this approach, the therapist would be able to take a lateral thinking approach and have a fresh perspective on the problem.

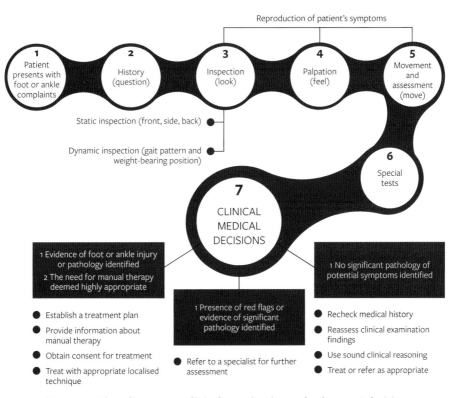

Figure 3.1 Flow diagram on clinical examination and subsequent decision making for patients presenting with foot and ankle pathology

Box 3.1 Important points that therapists need to cover during the history taking

- Age

- Profession and hobbies

- Involvement in sports and recreational exercises

- History of presenting complaint (e.g. type of trauma or pain and its onset or frequency)

- Specific mechanism of injury (if applicable)

- History of back or leg pain

- Presence of pain with other bodily joints (e.g. hip and knee)

- Pre-existing medical conditions (e.g. diabetes, vascular disease, arthritis, inflammatory arthropathy, neuropathy, cancer)

- Current and past medications

Adapted from Alazzawi et al. (2017)

Red flags

Table 3.1 Red flags for serious pathology in the foot and ankle complex

Condition	Signs and symptoms
Fractures	History of recent trauma such as a crush injury, ankle injury or a fall from height
	Pain, bruising or swelling on affected leg
	Persistent synovitis
	Point tenderness over involved tissues
	Inability to walk or bear weight on involved leg
Deep vein thrombosis	History of recent surgery
	Redness of the skin
	Swelling and tenderness in affected leg
	Pain intensified with walking or standing and reduced by elevation and rest
Peripheral neuropathy	Pricking, tingling or numbness in the lower limb
	Limb weakness

Septic arthritis	Fever, chills
	Recent bacterial infection, surgery or injection
	Severe, constant pain
	Systemically unwell such as unusual fatigue (malaise) or loss of appetite
	Coexisting immunosuppressive disorder
	Red, swollen joint with no history of trauma
Infection or neoplasm	Elevated body temperature
	Night sweating
	Sudden weight loss
Cancer	Unremitting pain
	Previous history of cancer
	Atypical symptoms with no history of a trauma
	Systematic symptoms such as fever, chills, malaise and weakness
	Unexplained weight loss
	Suspected malignancy or unexplained deformity, mass or swelling

Sources: Judd and Kim (2002); Ulmer (2002); Alazzawi et al. (2017); Kim (2019)

Inspection (look)

Inspection of patient's shoes, walking aids and orthoses

Before inspecting any patient presenting with foot or ankle complaints, the therapist should first examine the patient's shoes to ascertain whether they are commercial or custom-made. If the shoes are custom-made, the therapist should ask the patient about the specific foot or ankle deformity for which they have been designed (Alazzawi *et al.*, 2017). The therapist should then assess the wear pattern of the shoes, which normally involves the outer corner of the heel. Different wear patterns in the patient's shoes may give clues about the existence of any gait or rotational abnormalities (see Figures 3.2–3.4). Patients with shoe wear on the lateral border often have a supination deformity, whereas those with a pronation deformity (e.g., pes planus deformity) show more medial wear (Young *et al.*, 2005; Coughlin *et al.*, 2013). Always compare one side to the other. If there is no sign of wear in the patient's shoes, this may simply suggest the use of new or unused footwear. Finally, inspect inside the patient's shoes for insoles. Ask the patient whether they prefer any specific type of insoles and if the insoles are self-bought or professional recommended (Davies and Blundell, 2011; Bhatia and Aziz, 2020).

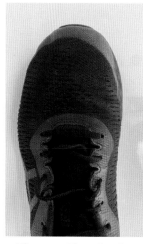
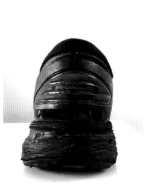
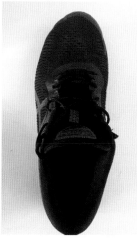

Figure 3.2 Shoe showing signs of left bunion

Figure 3.3 Left shoe of patient who has overpronation back

Figure 3.4 Left shoe overpronation full shoe

Note whether the patient has brought any walking aid or is using any orthosis. If a walking aid is present in the examination room, the therapist should inspect its type, on which side it is held and whether its height is right for the patient. The patient should also be asked to walk with and without their walking aids if possible. If orthoses are used, then they should be noted as seen, detailing their types and any hinges (if present). It should also be ascertained whether the use of orthoses is corrective or accommodative (Bensoussan *et al.*, 2008; Bhatia and Aziz, 2020).

From the front

In the first instance, the manual therapist should ask the patient to stand up with legs together, if possible. The therapist should then carefully assess the lower limbs as a whole and inspect the following in a logical order:

- The general alignment of both limbs, including leg length and rotational profile, to determine if there is an inequality in leg length.

- The alignment of the spine to rule out the presence of scoliosis and any pelvic obliquity.

- The knee joint alignment for varus (bow-leg) or valgus (knock-knee) deformities.

- The thigh or calf muscles for any signs of wasting.

- The plantar aspect of the sole for ecchymosis (bruising), which is indicative of Lisfranc injuries.

- The shape of the foot, in particular the width of the forefoot, to see whether the toes have any deformities such as hallux valgus or varus and claw toes.

- Between the toes for any signs of skin breakdown or active infection.

- The state of the skin for the presence of scar, ulcer, swelling, skin irritation, skin discoloration, callosities (skin thickening), loss of hair, varicosities (enlarged, tortuous veins) and active infection. If there are active or healed scars and/or ulcers, note their depth, size and location, and see how well they are healing or have healed (Davies and Blundell, 2011; Bhatia and Aziz, 2020).

Notes

- Hallux valgus refers to a condition in which the hallux deviates laterally (more than 10–15°) from the midline, while hallux varus causes the hallux to deviate medially away from the first metatarsal bone.

- The cavovarus deformity refers to a foot condition in which the arch is abnormally high while the heel slants inward.

- Claw toes are another common deformity of the foot that usually results from abnormal neurology. In this condition, the toes bend into a claw-like shape.

From the side

Viewing from the side, the manual therapist should inspect the following:

- The medial longitudinal arch, to assess whether there is any pes planus (flat arch) or pes cavus (high arch) (see Figures 3.5 and 3.6).

- The medial heel pad, which is normally not visible from the front. If the heel pad is seen, this is often referred to as a 'peek a boo' sign and represents cavovarus deformity (Coughlin *et al.*, 2013).

- The symmetry between both sides to rule out a false-positive 'peek a boo' sign.

- The hallux or lesser toes for any deformities such as hallux valgus or varus, hammer toes (flexion of the proximal interphalangeal joint), mallet toe (flexion of the distal interphalangeal joint) or claw toes.

- The position of the first ray to see if it is normal or hypermobile/hypomobile. Hypermobility of the first ray can be suggestive of plantar fasciitis, metatarsus adductus or hallux valgus, whereas hypomobility may increase the risk of fat pad ulceration in patients with diabetes (Papaliodis *et al.*, 2014).

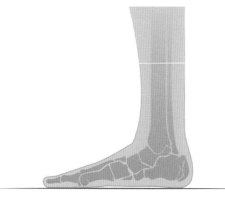

Figure 3.5 Flattening of medial longitudinal arch – pes planus

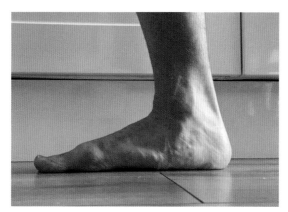

Figure 3.6 Flattening of medial longitudinal arch – pes planus

From the back

- Inspect the ankle joint for subtle swelling or any bony bumps (e.g. calcaneal boss). If the ankle is swollen, a visible blurring can be seen at the sharp outline of the Achilles tendon.

- Note the position of the heel. Unless there is any deformity, it will normally be in a neutral position (see Figure 3.7).

- Look for the 'too many toes' sign (Figure 3.8). Normally, only the fifth and fourth toes can be seen from behind. However, if more toes are visible, this can be suggestive of an increased heel valgus angle (Papaliodis *et al.*, 2014; Alazzawi *et al.*, 2017).

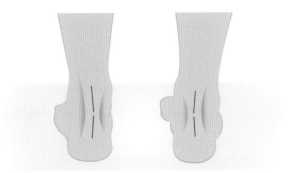

Figure 3.7 Normal valgus alignment of the hindfoot from the back

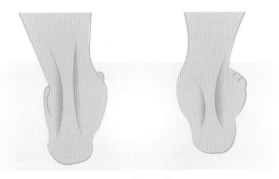

Figure 3.8 Hindfoot alignment

The left foot shows about 15° of valgus hindfoot alignment. 'Too many toes' sign – the right foot showing three toes. The right foot also shows mild medial bulging.

Dynamic inspection: gait assessment

The patient's gait needs to be evaluated during the clinical examination to note whether there is any deviation in normal gait pattern. The patient should be asked to walk a few steps away from the therapist, then turn around and walk directly back to observe the gait from both sides. Subtle gait abnormalities are usually unmasked while walking faster, so therapists should ask the patient to walk as needed, unless it is causing undue discomfort (Young *et al.*, 2005; Davies and Blundell, 2011).

What to inspect?

- Observe the rhythm, symmetry and cadence of the gait to check whether there is any deviation that may correlate with the abnormal gait patterns described in Chapter 2.

- Inspect the spine, hip, knee and ankle movements to assess if there is a shoulder or pelvic tilt or ankle stiffness.

- Note any abnormalities in the motion of any segment (e.g. arm swing, stride length).

The therapist should also ask the patient to walk on their heels, toes and lateral and medial borders. Table 3.2 shows the correlation between muscle weakness and different gait patterns (heels, toes, lateral and medial foot walking).

Table 3.2 Implications for muscle weakness in different gait patterns

Gait type examination	Assessment (involved muscle)	Implications for muscle weakness
Heel walking	Ankle dorsiflexor strength (tibialis anterior muscle)	L4 or L5 nerve injury or an L4 radiculopathy
Tiptoe walking	Ankle plantar flexor strength (the gastrocnemius-soleus complex)	Achilles tendon injury or sciatic or tibial nerve dysfunction
Lateral walking	Inversion strength (tibialis posterior muscle)	Tibial nerve dysfunction
Medial walking	Eversion strength (peroneal muscles)	Superficial peroneal nerve injury or dysfunction

Adapted from Young et al. (2005)

Note: The assessment of gait should be carried out methodically, starting from bottom to top or vice versa. The therapist must take the time needed to properly assess the patient's gait while they walk on all aspects of the foot.

Palpation (feel)

The goal of palpation should be to identify areas of pain, swelling, warmth, tenderness and tenosynovitis. Manual therapists should palpate the foot and ankle in an orderly manner so that all the parts are examined (Loudon *et al.*, 2008; Bhatia and Aziz, 2020).

We recommend doing the following during palpation:

- Ask the patient to identify any areas that are painful or highly tender so that undue discomfort can be avoided during examination.

- Assess the skin temperature of one side and then compare it to the other side. An increase in temperature may indicate Charcot arthropathy, while a decrease may be suggestive of peripheral vascular disease.

- Start the palpation from the proximal areas of the foot and then move to the distal parts (e.g. starting at the proximal fibula and then to the distal fibula). Palpate every part of the foot and ankle, including the joint lines, Achilles, tibialis and peroneal tendons, medial, lateral and deltoid ligaments, medial and lateral malleolus, extensors and other flexors, and plantar fascia (Alazzawi *et al.*, 2017).

Movement assessment (move)

Movement assessment of the foot and ankle is the last stage of the physical examination that includes the basics of look, feel and move. Similar to inspection and palpation, this should also be carried out in an orderly manner, starting proximally and moving distally. Therapists should assess both active and passive ranges of motion (ROMs). However, because the foot and ankle complex comprises many joints, the assessment can be deceptive. For example, stiffness in a particular joint may be masked by the adjacent joints. Hence, to correctly examine each joint, therapists should stabilise the adjacent joints with their other hand and compare the results to the contralateral side (Norkin and White, 2009; Davies and Blundell, 2011; Gross *et al.*, 2015).

Ankle joint movement

- **Active ROM assessment:** Ask the patient to carry out ankle dorsiflexion and plantarflexion. Measure the ROMs and compare them with the normal ROMs mentioned in Table 3.3.

- **Passive ROM assessment:** Grip the heel with the palm of one hand, hold the lower limb slightly above the ankle with the other hand, rest the sole on the forearm and then move downward and upward. Perform the measurements (see Figure 3.9).

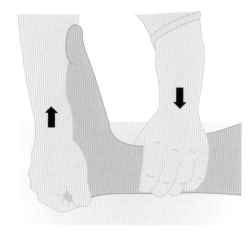

Figure 3.9 Passive dorsiflexion of the ankle

Subtalar joint movement

The subtalar joint allows the inversion and eversion of the ankle. The therapist should do the following to assess the active and passive ROMs of this joint:

- **Active ROM assessment:** Ask the patient to perform inversion and eversion movements. Measure the ROMs to check whether they are within the normal range cited in Table 3.3.

- **Passive ROM assessment:** Place the index finger and thumb of one hand over the talar neck, hold the heel with the palm of the other hand, then move the heel in medial and lateral directions to test for inversion and eversion, respectively (see Figure 3.10).

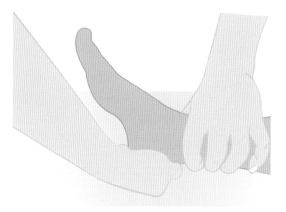

Figure 3.10 Passive subtalar joint movement

Table 3.3 Possible causes for laxity or restriction in ankle ROM

Movements	Normal ROM	Possible reasons for an increase or decrease in ROM
Dorsiflexion	0–20°	Achilles tendon tightness, anterior ankle impingement
Plantarflexion	0–45°	Anterior capsule tightness, posterior impingement
Inversion	0–35°	Lateral ligament laxity or injury, stiffness in joint capsules
Eversion	0–15°	Medial ligament (deltoid) injury, stiffness in joint capsules

Adapted from Alazzawi et al. (2017)

Midfoot movement

The following manoeuvres assess the talonavicular joint, which enables the forefoot to supinate and pronate on the hindfoot (see Figure 3.11).

- Place one hand over the talar neck, stabilising the talus with the thumb.

- Use the other hand to move the forefoot to its full range of motion.

- Check whether the forefoot maintains a neutral position and is in alignment with the hindfoot.

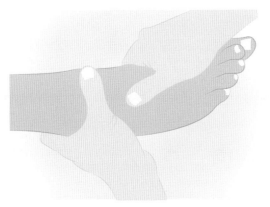

Figure 3.11 The talonavicular joint assessment

Forefoot movement

Assessment of movement for each forefoot joint should be done separately. The ROM of the first metatarsophalangeal joint should be assessed if arthritis is suspected in the patient. Perform the following manoeuvres to assess this joint:

- Support the first metatarsal with one hand and then move the hallux to its full ROM with the other.

- Note whether pain is elicited with maximum plantarflexion and dorsiflexion. Painful impingement at the extremes of movement is suggestive of dorsal osteophytes.

- Apply axial pressure over the joint, grinding it with slight circular movements. If there is pain and crepitus, the joint is probably arthritic.

Special tests

Single heel-raise test

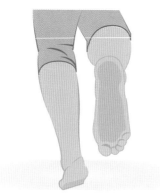 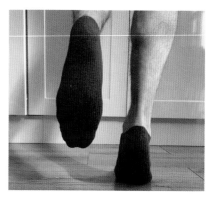

Procedure

- The patient stands on the test limb only, with the knee extended.

- The examiner asks the patient to plantarflex the ankle and raise the heel from the floor, standing on their toes.

Positive sign: absence of heel inversion during plantarflexion.

Interpretation: posterior tibial tendon dysfunction.

Anterior drawer test

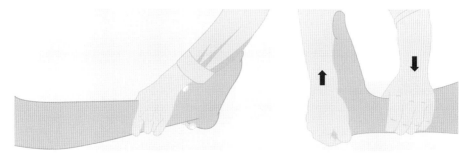

Procedure

- The patient lies prone on the table, with the ankle in a neutral position and the foot in 20° of plantarflexed position.

- The examiner stabilises the distal tibia with one hand and applies an anterior force to the calcaneus (heel) with the other hand.

Positive sign: increased anterior translation compared with the contralateral side.

Interpretation: compromised anterior talofibular ligament.

Talar tilt test

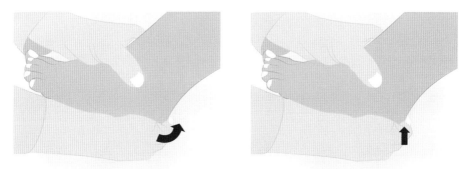

Procedure

- The patient is seated, with the ankle unsupported and the foot in 10–20° of plantarflexed position.

- The examiner stabilises the distal lower leg, just proximal to the medial malleolus, with one hand and applies an inversion force to the hindfoot with the other hand.

- The examiner tilts the talus side to side during inversion of the foot.

Positive sign: increased joint laxity or increased talar tilt compared to the other side.

Interpretation: compromised calcaneofibular ligament.

Thompson test

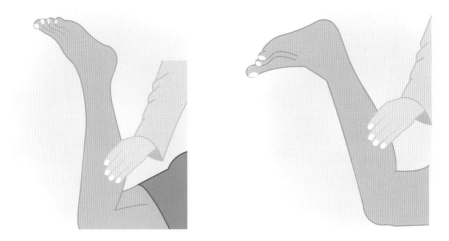

Procedure

- The patient lies prone, with the knee bent to 90°.

- The examiner squeezes the calf muscle and checks if the ankle plantarflexes.

Positive sign: absence of ankle plantarflexion.

Interpretation: Achilles tendon rupture.

References

Alazzawi, S., Sukeik, M., King, D. and Vemulapalli, K. (2017) Foot and ankle history and clinical examination: A guide to everyday practice. *World Journal of Orthopedics* 8, 1, 21–29.

Bensoussan, L., Viton, J.M., Barotsis, N. and Delarque, A. (2008) Evaluation of patients with gait abnormalities in physical and rehabilitation medicine settings. *Journal of Rehabilitation Medicine* 4, 7, 497–507.

Bhatia, M. and Aziz, S. (2020) Clinical Examination of the Foot and Ankle (Basic and Surface Anatomy) with Special Tests. In K.M. Iyer and W.S. Khan (eds) *Orthopedics of the Upper and Lower Limb.* Springer.

Chinn, L. and Hertel, J. (2010) Rehabilitation of ankle and foot injuries in athletes. *Clinics in Sports Medicine* 29, 1, 157–167.

Coughlin, M.J., Saltzman, C.L. and Mann, R.A. (2013) *Mann's Surgery of the Foot and Ankle E-Book: Expert Consult-Online.* Elsevier Health Sciences.

Davies, H. and Blundell, C. (2011) Clinical examination of the foot and ankle. *Orthopaedics and Trauma* 25, 4, 287–292.

Ferguson, R., Culliford, D., Prieto-Alhambra, D., Pinedo-Villanueva, R. *et al.* (2019) Encounters for foot and ankle pain in UK primary care: A population-based cohort study of CPRD data. *British Journal of General Practice* 69, 683, e422–e429.

Gross, J.M., Fetto, J. and Rosen, E. (2015) *Musculoskeletal Examination.* John Wiley & Sons.

Hartley, A. and Robinson, M.M. (1995) Book review: Practical Joint Assessment: Lower Quadrant: A Sports Medicine Manual. *Advanced Emergency Nursing Journal* 17, 2, 64–66.

Hunt, K.J., Hurwit, D., Robell, K., Gatewood, C., Botser, I.B. and Matheson, G. (2017) Incidence and epidemiology of foot and ankle injuries in elite collegiate athletes. *The American Journal of Sports Medicine* 45, 2, 426–433.

Judd, D.B. and Kim, D.H. (2002) Foot fractures frequently misdiagnosed as ankle sprains. *American Family Physician* 66, 5, 785–794.

Kim, Y.J. (2019) Red flag rules for knee and lower leg differential diagnosis. *Annals of Translational Medicine* 7, Suppl 7, S250.

Loudon, J.K., Swift, M. and Bell, S. (2008) *The Clinical Orthopedic Assessment Guide.* Human Kinetics.

Luciano, A.D.P. and Lara, L.C.R. (2012) Epidemiological study of foot and ankle injuries in recreational sports. *Acta Ortopedica Brasileira* 20, 6, 339–342.

Norkin, C.C. and White, D.J. (2009) *Measurement of Joint Motion: A Guide to Goniometry.* FA Davis.

Ohm, F., Vogel, D., Sehner, S., Wijnen-Meijer, M. and Harendza, S. (2013) Details acquired from medical history and patients' experience of empathy – two sides of the same coin. *BMC Medical Education* 13, 1, 1–7.

Papaliodis, D.N., Vanushkina, M.A., Richardson, N.G. and DiPreta, J.A. (2014) The foot and ankle examination. *Medical Clinics* 98, 2, 181–204.

Reissig, J., Bitterman, A. and Lee, S. (2017) Common foot and ankle injuries: What not to miss and how best to manage. *Journal of Osteopathic Medicine* 117, 2, 98–104.

Seitz, T., Raschauer, B., Längle, A.S. and Löffler-Stastka, H. (2019) Competency in medical history taking – the training physicians' view. *Wiener Klinische Wochenschrift* 131, 1, 17–22.

Ulmer, T. (2002) The clinical diagnosis of compartment syndrome of the lower leg: Are clinical findings predictive of the disorder? *Journal of Orthopaedic Trauma* 16, 8, 572–577.

Young, C.C., Niedfeldt, M.W., Morris, G.A. and Eerkes, K.J. (2005) Clinical examination of the foot and ankle. *Primary Care: Clinics in Office Practice* 32, 1, 105–132.

Chapter 4

Musculoskeletal Conditions of the Foot and Ankle

The foot and ankle are affected by a broad range of conditions, from simple bunion deformity to ankle sprains or tendon ruptures. Over the past decades, these conditions have become a major public health concern because of their increasing incidence and subsequent detrimental effects on patients' daily activity and quality of life (Rao *et al.*, 2012). The burden of these problems is likely to increase, as the number of older people is increasing in the general population. Studies have suggested that foot pain affects about 20–40% of people aged 45 years and older (Menz *et al.*, 2010), while ankle pain has been reported in around 15% of adults of the same age group (Thomas *et al.*, 2011). In total, foot and ankle conditions account for roughly 10% of all consultations in primary care for musculoskeletal problems (Walsh *et al.*, 2019). Hence, there is a need to understand the predisposing factors that may lead to foot and ankle problems.

From a broader perspective, the primary causative factor for foot and ankle conditions can be their inherent structural and functional complexities. The foot and ankle include a total of 28 bones and 33 joints stabilised by an interconnected network of muscles, nerves, ligaments and tendons. These structures also take part in weight-bearing; thus, an injury or problem in any of these structures of the foot or ankle can have a cascading effect on adjacent structures. This may ultimately give rise to additional problems or other symptoms (Towers *et al.*, 2003).

Functionally, the major causes of foot and ankle injuries include involvement in high-impact activities such as running and jumping, long-term degenerative changes in joints and development of overuse issues due to repetitive microtrauma or continued wear and tear (Reissig *et al.*, 2017). On the other hand, the foot and ankle can undergo structural changes over time through activities of daily living. This can eventually reshape the feet and lead to several deformities and pathologies. Furthermore, the foot and ankle are frequently infected by common pathogens such as bacteria, fungi, viruses, prions and parasites when there is a break in the skin. Systemic illnesses such as diabetes can also lead to bacterial colonisation and eventual diabetic foot infections (Anakwenze *et al.*, 2012).

Taken together, in light of the above, it is of critical importance for manual therapists to thoroughly assess a patient when there is an ankle or foot problem. This chapter therefore provides an overview of the common musculoskeletal conditions of the foot and ankle with an emphasis on trauma- or sports-related injuries.

Ankle sprain

Ankle sprain is the most common injury to the ankle linked to both short-term and long-term disability. It involves stretching the strong ankle ligaments beyond their limits and, possibly, tearing them. Of the ligamentous structures present in the ankle, the lateral ligamentous complex is the most commonly sprained structure (Struijs and Kerkhoffs, 2010). Lateral ligament injuries account for about 85% of all ankle sprains, whereas spraining of the medial ligament complex and the tibiofibular syndesmosis comprises approximately 5% and 10% of all ankle injuries, respectively (Hodler *et al.*, 2021).

The severity of ankle sprains can be graded into three categories:

- **Grade I sprains** include mild or minor stretching of the ligament complex. The ankle joint stays stable and no tearing of ligaments occurs.

- **Grade II sprains** involve incomplete or partial tearing of one or more ligaments (e.g. an isolated tear of the anterior talofibular ligament (ATFL)). The ankle joint becomes mildly unstable.

- **Grade III sprains** are those in which complete rupturing of the ligaments occurs. The ankle joint becomes completely unstable.

High-risk group: Individuals who participate in forceful athletic activities, which require rapid shifting of movement, such as running and jumping sports. However, ankle sprains affect both general people and athletes alike, and the spraining can occur even from simple activities such as walking down the street (Chen *et al.*, 2019).

Rate of incidence: One injury per 10,000 individuals a day (Struijs and Kerkhoffs, 2010).

Lateral ankle sprains

Lateral ankle sprains are usually caused by a combination of inversion and adduction stresses, resulting from abnormal subtalar inversion and talocrural plantarflexion. These injuries often lead to tears of the ATFL either in isolation or in combination with the calcaneofibular ligament (CFL). However, isolated ATFL tears are more common and account for about 70% of all lateral ankle sprains (Fong *et al.*, 2007).

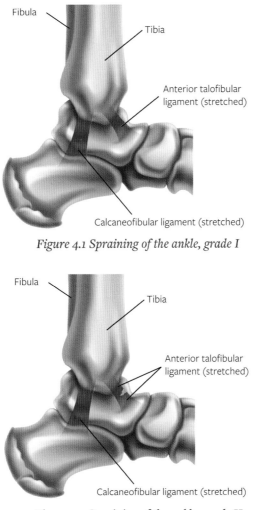

Fibula

Tibia

Anterior talofibular ligament (stretched)

Calcaneofibular ligament (stretched)

Figure 4.1 Spraining of the ankle, grade I

Fibula

Tibia

Anterior talofibular ligament (stretched)

Calcaneofibular ligament (stretched)

Figure 4.2 Spraining of the ankle, grade II

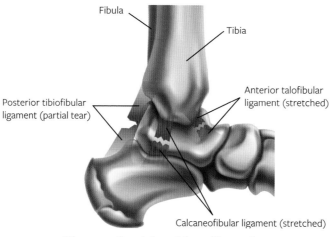

Figure 4.3 Spraining of the ankle, grade III

Associated conditions/injuries

- Anterolateral impingement
- Osteochondral defects
- Peroneal tenosynovitis
- Syndesmotic tear
- Medial/deltoid ligament complex injury
- Bifurcate ligament injury
- Fractures
- Complex regional pain syndrome

Clinical presentation

- Pain, mild to severe swelling, bruising
- Ankle joint instability and stiffness
- History of ankle twisting or rolling to the side during normal or athletic activities
- Inability to weight-bear on the affected foot
- Localised tenderness in the area of ATFL
- Repeated bouts of 'giving way' of the lateral ankle

- Pain at ankle dorsiflexion and restriction in range of motion

- Decreased ankle proprioception and problem in balance control

Table 4.1 Classification of different grades of ankle sprains and their clinical relevance

Grade	I	II	III
Pain and swelling on palpation	Mild	Moderate	Severe
Ecchymosis	Mild	Mild to moderate	Severe
Tenderness at the affected ligament	Mild	Moderate to severe	Severe
Sprain type	Stretching of the ATFL/CFL	Partial tearing of either the AFTL or both the AFTL and the CFL	Complete tearing of both the AFTL and the CFL
Ankle stability	Stable	Mild to moderate instability	Mechanical instability
Movement and function	Slight or no loss of motion and function	Some loss of motion and function	Loss of motion and function
Anterior drawer test	Negative	Positive	Positive
Talar tilt test	Negative	Negative	Positive

Adapted from Wolfe et al. (2001); Iyer and Khan (2013)

Achilles tendinopathy

Achilles tendinopathy is a non-rupture injury of the Achilles (calcaneal) tendon. It is a common overuse injury that often results from repeated trauma or stress to the tendon. This can lead to a more serious injury over time where the tendon may rupture, either partially or fully (Abat *et al.*, 2018). The condition is also described by some as tendinitis, tendinosis, tenosynovitis or paratenonitis. However, Maffulli (1998) suggested that the correct terminology for this condition should be tendinopathy due to its histopathology and clinical signs. The suffix 'osis' is indicative of a degenerative process, while 'itis' is indicative of an inflammatory disorder. As it is not always clear whether the condition is purely degenerative or inflammatory in nature, the terminology of tendinopathy is more appropriate.

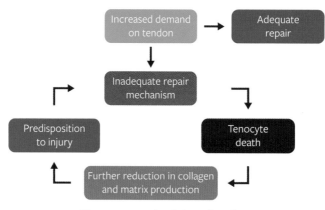

Figure 4.4 Tendon injury flowchart

Achilles tendinopathy is classified into two categories based on its anatomical location. The first is insertional (at the calcaneus tendon junction) and the second is non-insertional (2–3 inches from the proximal insertion on to the calcaneus) (Almekinders and Temple, 1998).

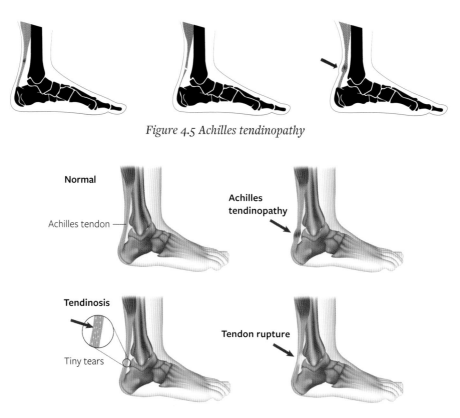

Figure 4.5 Achilles tendinopathy

Figure 4.6 Achilles tendon problems

Anatomy

The Achilles tendon is a long tendon that attaches the muscle bellies of the triceps surae muscles (lateral and medial heads of the gastrocnemius and the soleus) to the posterior surface of the calcaneus. The plantaris muscle can, in some individuals, insert directly on to the posterior surface of the calcaneus or merge its fibres with the calcaneal tendon. The plantaris muscle, which is often thought of as an obsolete accessory muscle, is absent in around 7–20% of the population (Spina, 2007). This may be detrimental to those who are missing the muscle, as its tendon is an excellent source for a graft (Simpson *et al.*, 1991).

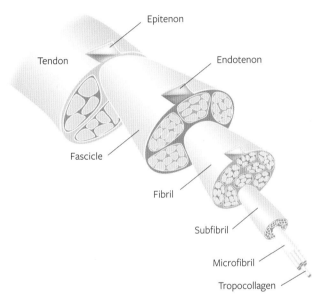

Figure 4.7 Tendon structure

Signs and symptoms

One of the major signs of tendinopathy is morning pain, which is characterised by pain and stiffness on waking up.

Other signs and symptoms include:

- pain and stiffness
- tenderness
- change in shape (tendon outline)
- impaired walking

- impaired performance

- crepitus

- swelling (less common).

Risk factors

There are multiple risk factors for developing an Achilles tendinopathy, both intrinsic and extrinsic in nature (Li and Hua, 2016). These include:

- age

- poor mobility and flexibility

- poor conditioning

- inappropriate footwear

- sudden increase in training load or mileage

- excessive hill running

- anatomic predisposition

- obesity

- corticosteroid use

- hypertension

- diabetes.

Diagnosis

To accurately diagnose Achilles tendinopathy, a full subjective and objective examination should be carried out.

Observation and palpation: Assess the patient's standing posture and ability to walk or sit to stand. Assessment should be made for asymmetry between the affected and non-affected tendons, along with any signs of muscle atrophy, oedema or swelling.

Movement and muscles: Assess the active and passive range of motions of the muscles and joints of the lower leg. The passive length of the muscles should also be assessed along with their strengths. Dynamic testing may be used in the form of single-leg hops or heel-raise tests to assess the muscle endurance of both legs.

Special tests: A number of tests can be conducted to detect possible tendinopathy, either through a subjective evaluation (self-reported pain or reporting of morning stiffness) or via palpatory assessments (tendon thickening, crepitus, the arc sign). Some tendon-loading tests may also be performed such as the Royal London Hospital test, single-leg hops, single heel-raise test and passive dorsiflexion stretch.

Achilles rupture

Achilles tendon rupture (ATR) is one of the most common tendon pathologies caused by overuse stress or sudden trauma (Shamrock and Varacallo, 2021). ATR is common in the physically active populations, especially among runners and athletes. However, anyone with no prior history of injuries can also have an ATR. It can occur through an acute injury while participating in sports or by way of tendinopathies from a chronic background (Klatte-Schulz *et al.*, 2018).

Signs and symptoms

The most common sign of an Achilles rupture is a sudden onset of pain in the lower leg and heel, which is generally a sharp stabbing pain. A 'pop' may also be heard when the tendon ruptures.

Other symptoms may include:

- swelling – around the heel and ankle
- decreased ability to plantarflex the foot
- decreased ability to bear weight
- impaired gait
- increased passive dorsiflexion
- inability to raise heel
- positive outcome on Thompson test.

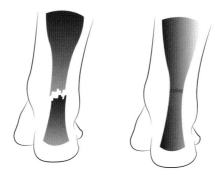

Figure 4.8 Achilles rupture

Risk factors

- **Age:** The average age of a patient suffering from a rupture is 30–40.

- **Gender:** Males are five times more likely to suffer a rupture than women.

- **Recreational sports:** Achilles tendon injuries occur more often during sports that involve running, jumping and sudden dynamic changes in direction.

- **Change in intensity of training:** This may occur due to a sharp increase in the volume or intensity of training, such as a steep increase in mileage of a runner, or the introduction of intermediate or advanced plyometrics.

- **Steroid injections:** This course of medication can weaken tendons and has been associated with Achilles tendon ruptures.

- **Long-term antibiotic use:** Fluoroquinolone antibiotics, such as ciprofloxacin (Cipro) or levofloxacin (Levaquin), increase the risk of Achilles tendon rupture.

- **Obesity:** Excess weight puts more strain on the tendon.

Diagnosis

Diagnosis of ATR should be made through a comprehensive subjective and objective examination.

Observation and palpation: Assess the patient's standing posture, ability to walk or sit to stand. With the tendon being easily palpable, assessment should be made for the tone of the tendon and its surrounding musculature as well as for a possible 'gap' at the site of the rupture. Care should be taken to assess any signs of oedema, muscle atrophy and bruising.

Movement and muscles: Assess the active and passive range of motions of the muscles and joints of the lower leg. The passive length of the muscles should also be assessed along with their strengths. Care should be taken when assessing foot plantarflexion as this movement can be highly painful for the patient.

Special tests: The Thompson test may be used during the physical examination to assess the integrity of the Achilles tendon. However, as this is a provocative test, appropriate caution should be exercised so as not to cause undue pain and stress to the patient. Hence, the patient's SIN (severity, irritability and nature) factor should also be evaluated.

Stress fractures

Stress fractures of the foot and ankle are the most common type of bone injuries diagnosed on imaging. They are characterised by a small crack or break in the bone or a deep bone bruise. Most stress fractures usually occur from repetitive trauma to a bone over time. However, a key difference from a sudden traumatic fracture is that the bone does not displace from its position in a stress fracture (Asano *et al.*, 2014; Welck *et al.*, 2017).

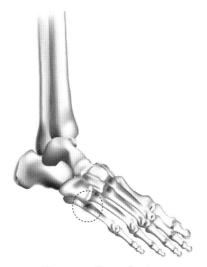

Figure 4.9 Stress fracture

There are two types of stress fractures.

Fatigue-type fractures are often caused by sudden abnormal stress on a normal bone. This type of fracture is more common in athletes who participate in running sports such as foot races, football, basketball, cricket or tennis. Such fractures usually occur from overuse of the foot and ankle. Because athletic people expose their weight-bearing bones and supporting muscles to frequent, repetitive motion, the bones get little time to undergo healing or remodelling. As a result, when there is a sudden change in physical activity, those weakened bones become vulnerable to stress fractures (Sonoda *et al.*, 2003; Hodler *et al.*, 2021).

Insufficiency-type fractures happen when everyday activities lead to a crack in an abnormally weak bone. Such weakening of bones usually occurs from an underlying condition (e.g. osteoporosis) that decreases bone strength and density over time. As a result, these bones lack the durability to bear normal impact forces and thus are vulnerable to stress fractures even from relatively low-impact activities such as walking. This type of fracture is more common in female athletes than male athletes. The most likely reason for this is a condition called the 'female athlete triad' (Asano *et al.*, 2014).

Common locations

Stress fractures can occur at any bone of the foot and ankle. The most commonly fractured bones include:

- the metatarsal bones
- the calcaneus (heel bone)
- the navicular
- the sesamoids
- the tibia and fibula.

Less common sites of stress fractures at the ankle and foot are:

- the medial malleolus
- the talus
- the cuneiform and cuboid bones.

Signs and symptoms

- Pain, swelling or possibly bruising at the site of injury.

- Pain begins and intensifies with normal activities but diminishes with rest.

- Pain worsens with weight-bearing on the affected foot.

- Tenderness on the affected bone with palpation.

- Pain is constant during everyday walking.

Diagnosis

Radiographs are most commonly used to diagnose stress fractures. However, because X-rays are less sensitive to identifying small cracks in bones, more sensitive testing such as magnetic resonance imaging (MRI) or bone scanning is often recommended to detect early signs of fracture (Hodler *et al.*, 2021).

Peroneal tendon disorders

Peroneal tendon disorders or pathologies are a common overuse injury causing lateral hindfoot pain and dysfunction. The peroneal tendons include two pero-neal muscles: peroneus brevis and peroneus longus. The superficial peroneal nerve innervates both muscles. The vascular supply to these muscles comes from the peroneal artery and the tibialis anterior artery (Davda *et al.*, 2017). Studies suggest that the peroneus brevis tears more often in isolation whereas the peroneus longus is torn less frequently. The peroneus longus often tears at the cuboid tunnel (Hallinan *et al.*, 2019).

Peroneal tendon pathologies are broadly divided into three categories:

- peroneal tendinitis and tenosynovitis

- peroneal subluxation or dislocation

- peroneal tendon splits or tears.

These pathologies usually occur as a result of excessive eversion and prona-tion. They are more common in athletes, especially among runners. Because runners' feet are often rolled outwards, friction between the tendon and bone occurs more frequently. When left untreated, peroneal tendon pathologies can cause severe ankle pain, foot deformity and significant functional problems (Sharma and Parekh, 2021).

Other conditions commonly associated with peroneal tendon pathologies include:

- cavovarus hindfoot alignment

- cavovalgus foot deformity

- ankle sprains

- chronic lateral ankle instability.

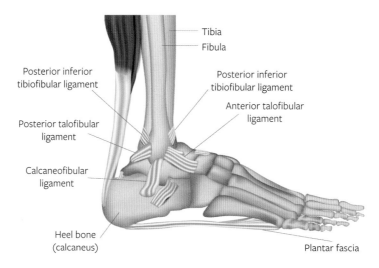

Figure 4.10 Lateral ankle ligaments

Peroneal tendinitis and tenosynovitis

Peroneal tendinitis simply refers to inflammation or irritation of the peroneal tendons. Tenosynovitis is tendinitis with inflammation at the synovial sheath that covers each peroneal tendon separately (DiGiovanni *et al.*, 2000; Heckman *et al.*, 2009).

Patients with peroneal tendinitis or tenosynovitis may present with the following symptoms:

- posterolateral ankle pain and swelling

- pain that intensifies with normal activities and lessens with rest

- pain when getting up in the morning

- tenderness overlying the peroneal tendons (posterior to the lateral malleolus)

- swelling and warmth along the sheath covering the peroneal tendons

- increased range of motion of the tendons, particularly around the fibula

- ankle instability during weight-bearing.

Peroneal subluxation or dislocation

Peroneal tendon subluxation or dislocation is a condition in which the superior peroneal retinaculum (SPR) is torn, stretched or avulsed. The SPR is a tough fibrous band that holds the peroneal tendons in place. However, recent studies also suggest an intrasheath, or internal, subluxation of the tendons in which the SPR remains intact (Heckman *et al.*, 2009; Davda *et al.*, 2017).

The mechanisms of tendon subluxation involve forced ankle dorsiflexion and hindfoot inversion, which results in strong reflex contraction of the peroneal tendons, causing injury to the SPR. As a result, one or both peroneal tendons displace from their normal position and slip over the lateral malleolus. The subluxation or dislocation of the tendons mostly occurs at the retromalleolar groove. In addition, of the two peroneal tendons, peroneus longus is more commonly affected by dislocation than the peroneus brevis (Selmani *et al.*, 2006; Hallinan *et al.*, 2019; Sharma and Parekh, 2021).

Signs and symptoms

- A painful snapping or popping sensation at the lateral ankle.

- Pain, swelling and ecchymosis below/behind the lateral malleolus.

- Pain with foot dorsiflexion and eversion.

- Marked tenderness and crepitus over the tendons.

- Sharp pain behind the outside ankle bone.

- Increased range of motion of the peroneal tendons.

- Ankle instability during weight-bearing.

Clinical presentation

SPR injuries can be classified into four grades using Oden's classification (Oden, 1987):

- **Grade I injuries** involve stripping of the retinaculum off the fibula, making a pouch for the subluxation of the tendons.

- **Grade II injuries** cause avulsion of the SPR and the fibrocartilaginous ridge from their posterior fibular attachment.

- **Grade III injuries** involve avulsion of a thin cortical fragment of the SPR from the fibula.

- **Grade IV injuries** are characterised by a tear of the SPR from its calcaneus attachment.

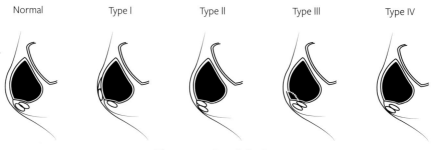

Figure 4.11 SPR injuries

Diagnosis

Peroneal tendon injuries are often misdiagnosed as lateral ankle ligament injuries. Hence, a thorough clinical examination of the foot and ankle is warranted to fully evaluate the injury. Special tests such as a Coleman block test and a compression test may be performed during the physical exam. Bilateral weight-bearing radiographs and other advanced imaging studies such as MRI and dynamic ultrasound should be performed to identify peroneal tendon instability (Davda *et al.*, 2017; Sharma and Parekh, 2021).

Plantar fasciitis

Plantar fasciitis is a degenerative disease of the plantar fascia, which causes stabbing pain in the heel and bottom of the foot. The cause of plantar fasciitis can be multifactorial, but it primarily occurs from overuse stress on the plantar fascia ligament. The condition most commonly affects the middle-aged population and athletic people; about 10% of individuals develop it at some stage during their lifetime (Lim *et al.*, 2016; Becker and Childress, 2018).

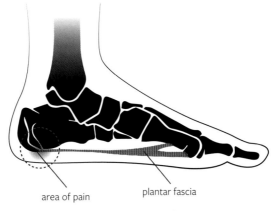

area of pain   plantar fascia

Figure 4.12 Plantar fasciitis

Clinical presentation

- Sharp localised pain at the medial side of the heel.

- Pain worsens in the morning while taking the first few steps but subsides with a short period of walking.

- Pain returns with prolonged weight-bearing activities such as running, walking or standing.

- Point tenderness from palpation over the plantar medial calcaneal tuberosity.

- Pain reproduces with passive foot dorsiflexion.

Risk factors

- Obesity.

- Leg-length inconsistency.

- Foot deformity such as pes planus or pes cavus.

- Reduced ankle dorsiflexion.

- Nerve entrapment syndrome.

- Calf muscle tightness.

- Excessive pronation.

- Over-training.

- Prolonged walking/standing.

- Using ill-fitting footwear.

Diagnosis

Plantar fasciitis is often diagnosed through history evaluation and physical examination. Imaging studies are usually not necessary; however, lateral weight-bearing radiographs and dynamic ultrasound can be helpful to conclusively exclude differentials (Buchanan and Kushner, 2017).

Lisfranc joint injuries

The Lisfranc tarsometatarsal construct is a very stable joint complex with articulations between metatarsal bases and distal tarsals supported by the Lisfranc ligament. This joint allows significant loading of the foot during the gait cycle. Lisfranc joint injury is relatively rare and accounts for only 0.2% of all fractures (Iyer and Khan, 2013). However, if an injury occurs to this joint, it can be significantly disabling and painful. The mechanisms of Lisfranc injury include both low-energy (indirect) and high-energy (direct) injuries. Low-energy Lisfranc injuries occur from axial force through the foot, while direct injuries often result from sudden, excessive force on the dorsum of the foot such as a fall from a height or a motor vehicle accident (Sands and Grose, 2004).

Lisfranc joint injury is often associated with a number of other injury patterns. These include:

- soft-tissue injuries

- sprains or ligamentous injuries

- vascular compromise

- fractures at the Lisfranc joint complex.

Diagnosis

Diagnosis of Lisfranc injuries requires a high degree of clinical suspicion to avoid misdiagnosis. Because about one-third of Lisfranc injuries are subtle, low-energy cases, bilateral weight-bearing radiographs are often used to diagnose these injuries (Reissig *et al.*, 2017). Clinicians should pay special attention to the first and second tarsometatarsal joints for abnormal widening (> 2 mm), and avulsion fracture. If X-rays are inconclusive to identify a suspected injury, an MRI and/or computed tomography (CT) scan should be performed as a second imaging modality (Raikin *et al.*, 2009).

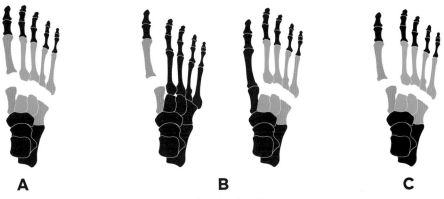

A   **B**   **C**

Figure 4.13 Hardcastle classification system

Foot and ankle pain presentation and possible differential diagnosis

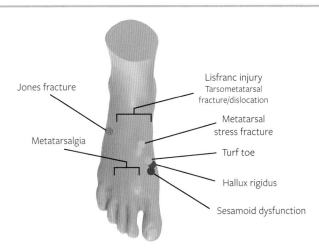

Figure 4.14 Anterior foot pain presentation and possible diagnosis

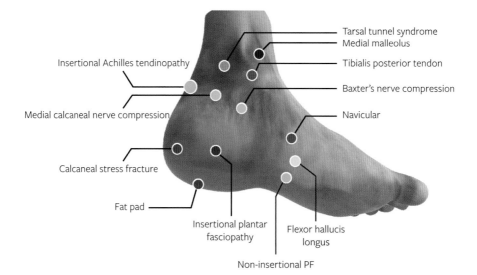

Figure 4.15 Medial foot pain presentation and possible diagnosis

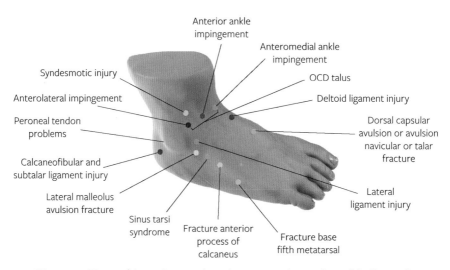

Figure 4.16 Lateral inversion sprain pain presentation and possible diagnosis

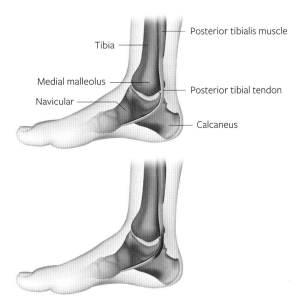

Figure 4.17 Posterior tibialis tendon dysfunction

References

Abat, F., Alfredson, H., Cucchiarini, M., Madry, H. *et al.* (2018) Current trends in tendinopathy: Consensus of the ESSKA basic science committee. Part II: treatment options. *Journal of Experimental Orthopaedics* 5, 1, 38.

Almekinders, L.C. and Temple, J.D. (1998) Etiology, diagnosis, and treatment of tendonitis: An analysis of the literature. *Medicine and Science in Sports and Exercise* 30, 8, 1183–1190.

Anakwenze, O.A., Milby, A.H., Gans, I., Stern, J.J., Levin, S.L. and Wapner, K.L. (2012) Foot and ankle infections: Diagnosis and management. *Journal of the American Academy of Orthopaedic Surgeons* 20, 11, 684–693.

Asano, L.Y.J., Duarte, A. and Silva, A.P.S. (2014) Stress fractures in the foot and ankle of athletes. *Revista da Associação Médica Brasileira* 60, 512–517.

Becker, B.A. and Childress, M.A. (2018) Common foot problems: Over-the-counter treatments and home care. *American Family Physician* 98, 5, 298–303.

Buchanan, B.K. and Kushner, D. (2017) Plantar Fasciitis. StatPearls [Internet], www.ncbi.nlm. nih.gov/books/NBK431073

Chen, E.T., McInnis, K.C. and Borg-Stein, J. (2019) Ankle sprains: Evaluation, rehabilitation, and prevention. *Current Sports Medicine Reports* 18, 6, 217–223.

Davda, K., Malhotra, K., O'Donnell, P., Singh, D. and Cullen, N. (2017) Peroneal tendon disorders. *EFORT Open Reviews* 2, 6, 281–292.

DiGiovanni, B.F., Fraga, C.J., Cohen, B.E. and Shereff, M.J. (2000) Associated injuries found in chronic lateral ankle instability. *Foot and Ankle International* 21, 10, 809–815.

Fong, D.T.P., Hong, Y., Chan, L.K., Yung, P.S.H. and Chan, K.M. (2007) A systematic review on ankle injury and ankle sprain in sports. *Sports Medicine* 37, 1, 73–94.

Hallinan, J.T.P.D., Wang, W., Pathria, M.N., Smitaman, E. and Huang, B.K. (2019) The peroneus longus muscle and tendon: A review of its anatomy and pathology. *Skeletal Radiology* 48, 9, 1329–1344.

Heckman, D.S., Gluck, G.S. and Parekh, S.G. (2009) Tendon disorders of the foot and ankle, part 1: Peroneal tendon disorders. *The American Journal of Sports Medicine* 37, 3, 614–625.

Hodler, J., Kubik-Huch, R.A. and von Schulthess, G.K. (2021) Ankle and Foot. In J. Hodler, R.A. Kubik-Huch and G.K. von Schulthess (eds) *Musculoskeletal Diseases 2021–2024: Diagnostic Imaging.* Springer.

Iyer, K.M. and Khan, W.S. (eds) (2013) *Orthopedics of the Upper and Lower Limb.* Springer.

Klatte-Schulz, F., Minkwitz, S., Schmock, A., Bormann, N. *et al.* (2018) Different Achilles tendon pathologies show distinct histological and molecular characteristics. *International Journal of Molecular Sciences* 19, 2, 404.

Li, H. and Hua, Y. (2016) Achilles tendinopathy: Current concepts about the basic science and clinical treatments. *BioMed Research International* 2016, 6492597.

Lim, A.T., How, C.H. and Tan, B. (2016) Management of plantar fasciitis in the outpatient setting. *Singapore Medical Journal* 57, 4, 168–170.

Maffulli, N. (1998) Overuse tendon conditions: Time to change a confusing terminology. *Arthroscopy: The Journal of Arthroscopic & Related Surgery* 14, 8, 840–843.

Menz, H.B., Jordan, K.P., Roddy, E. and Croft, P.R. (2010) Musculoskeletal foot problems in primary care: What influences older people to consult? *Rheumatology* 49, 11, 2109–2116.

Oden, R.R. (1987) Tendon injuries about the ankle resulting from skiing. *Clinical Orthopaedics and Related Research* 1987, 216, 63–69.

Raikin, S.M., Elias, I., Dheer, S., Besser, M.P., Morrison, W.B. and Zoga, A.C. (2009) Prediction of midfoot instability in the subtle Lisfranc injury: Comparison of magnetic resonance imaging with intraoperative findings. *Journal of Bone and Joint Surgery* 91, 4, 892–899.

Rao, S., Riskowski, J.L. and Hannan, M.T. (2012) Musculoskeletal conditions of the foot and ankle: Assessments and treatment options. *Best Practice and Research: Clinical Rheumatology* 26, 3, 345–368.

Reissig, J., Bitterman, A. and Lee, S. (2017) Common foot and ankle injuries: What not to miss and how best to manage. *Journal of Osteopathic Medicine* 117, 2, 98–104.

Sands, A.K. and Grose, A. (2004) Lisfranc injuries. *Injury* 35, SB71–76.

Selmani, E., Gjata, V. and Gjika, E. (2006) Current concepts review: Peroneal tendon disorders. *Foot and Ankle International* 27, 3, 221–228.

Shamrock, A.G. and Varacallo, M. (2021) Achilles Tendon Rupture. StatPearls [Internet], www.ncbi.nlm.nih.gov/books/NBK430844

Sharma, A. and Parekh, S.G. (2021) Pathologies of the peroneals: A review. *Foot and Ankle Specialist* 14, 2, 170–177.

Simpson, S.L., Hertzog, M.S. and Barja, R.H. (1991) The plantaris tendon graft: An ultrasound study. *The Journal of Hand Surgery* 16, 4, 708–711.

Sonoda, N., Chosa, E., Totoribe, K. and Tajima, N. (2003) Biomechanical analysis for stress fractures of the anterior middle third of the tibia in athletes: Nonlinear analysis using a three-dimensional finite element method. *Journal of Orthopaedic Science* 8, 4, 505–513.

Spina, A.A. (2007) The plantaris muscle: Anatomy, injury, imaging, and treatment. *Journal of the Canadian Chiropractic Association* 51, 3, 158–165.

Struijs, P.A. and Kerkhoffs, G.M. (2010) Ankle sprain. *BMJ Clinical Evidence* 2010, 1115.

Thomas, M.J., Roddy, E., Zhang, W., Menz, H.B., Hannan, M.T. and Peat, G.M. (2011) The population prevalence of foot and ankle pain in middle and old age: A systematic review. *Pain* 152, 12, 2870–2880.

Towers, J.D., Deible, C.T. and Golla, S.K. (2003) Foot and ankle biomechanics. *Seminars in Musculoskeletal Radiology* 7, 1, 67–74.

Walsh, T.P., Ferris, L.R., Cullen, N.C., Bourke, J.L. *et al.* (2019) Management of musculoskeletal foot and ankle conditions prior to public-sector orthopaedic referral in South Australia. *Journal of Foot and Ankle Research* 12, 1, 1–9.

Welck, M.J., Hayes, T., Pastides, P., Khan, W. and Rudge, B. (2017) Stress fractures of the foot and ankle. *Injury* 48, 8, 1722–1726.

Wolfe, M.W., Uhl, T.L., Mattacola, C.G. and McCluskey, L.C. (2001) Management of ankle sprains. *American Family Physician* 63, 1, 93–104.

Chapter 5

Leg-Length Discrepancy – Myth or Real?

DR JAMES INKLEBARGER

Manual therapy is an alternative treatment approach in which therapists utilise their hands or a hands-on technique for the management of various musculo-skeletal conditions. The therapy has been proven to be an effective treatment option to reduce musculoskeletal pain and restore mobility, flexibility and balance (Lederman, 2005; Bialosky *et al.*, 2011). However, as with other medical therapies, things can be misinterpreted, misused and go wrong in the practice of manual therapy. There can be diagnostic errors with the task at hand, which may eventually lead to therapeutic errors (Cook, 2011). How often do we see therapists showing before and after pictures of the tiniest difference in the patient's leg length following the use of a technique to lengthen or reposition the pelvis? Is this old biomechanical paradigm of correcting anatomy still valid? Is it still a useful diagnostic tool?

Clinical practice errors in manual therapy also occur due to the lack of manual and/or cognitive skills, past experiences and current medical knowledge. Because manual therapists often apply some or a combination of different techniques, they can subject their patients to further injuries of varying magnitudes when these errors occur. Ultimately, these actions violate patients' trust in manual therapy. Hence, the goal of every aspiring manual therapist should be to provide the therapy in a way that minimises these errors and improves patient safety (Boyling and Jull, 2004; Cochran *et al.*, 2009).

In the management of ankle and foot pathology, a common clinical problem that may lead manual therapists to errors in practice is leg-length discrepancy (LLD) or anisomelia. LLD is a condition in which the paired legs have a noticeable inequality in length – that is, one leg is shorter or longer than the other. In most clinical settings, manual therapists often try to fix LLDs after assessing minute differences in leg length. Many do not even consider whether such inequalities between two legs are clinically relevant or whether the methods used are valid and reliable for LLD measurement. However, it is to be noted that there has been little consensus among researchers and clinicians regarding the magnitude of LLD necessary to be clinically significant, the effects of LLD on various musculoskeletal conditions, and the accuracy and reliability of measuring methods (Gurney, 2002; Khamis and Carmeli, 2017; Collebrusco *et al.*, 2020). Such inconsistencies in the literature require manual therapists to be more cautious when making a clinical decision about treating LLDs; unfortunately, the opposite is currently the reality in most manual therapy clinics. This chapter therefore provides an evidence-based overview of the assessment and treatment of LLD so that manual therapists can make more informed clinical decisions.

Leg-length discrepancies: to treat or not to treat?

Epidemiology

LLD affects around 40–70% of the population (Gurney, 2002). Although the prevalence and extent of LLD are not well established, it is frequently mentioned in the literature that about 90% of the normal population generally have a small degree of LLD – that is, less than 10 mm (Gordon and Davis, 2019). Up to now, two studies, a US study and a Swedish one, reported that ≥ 10 mm of LLD could be present in one-third of the population (Hellsing, 1988; Brady *et al.*, 2003). In addition, a French retrospective study found that more than 20 mm of LLD could affect one person in every 1000 (Guichet *et al.*, 1991).

Risks associated with LLD

LLD can lead to several pathological conditions by causing postural compensations. These include low back pain, flank pain, gait asymmetry, gonarthrosis, coxarthrosis, ankle joint contracture, discopathy, hip contracture, degenerative disorders of the lower limb, and muscle imbalances, to name a few (Gurney, 2002). The postural deformity and associated symptoms of LLD can significantly influence the function and quality of life of an affected person. These problems arising from LLD, however, largely depend on the degree of variance in leg-length inequality (Khamis and Carmeli, 2017; Vogt *et al.*, 2020).

Classification of LLD

LLD can be broadly categorised into two types: anatomical LLD and functional LLD.

Anatomical LLDs are those that result from an actual shortening of bony structures. People with this type of LLD often have a shortening of one limb between the hip (thigh bone) and the ankle joint compared to the other. Anatomical LLD can be congenital or acquired and primarily occurs either due to bone loss or from an epiphyseal plate injury (Hasler, 2000). Patients with congenital LLD usually have developmental abnormalities at birth or in childhood, which manifest with continuous slower growth of the affected limb compared with the normal one. Acquired anatomic LLDs, on the other hand, often occur later in life and can result from trauma, infections, fractures, surgical disorders or degenerative conditions (Knutson, 2005; Vogt *et al.*, 2020).

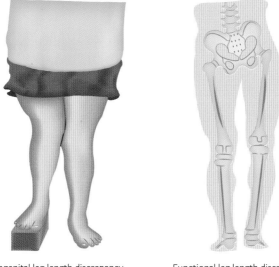

Congenital leg length discrepancy　　　Functional leg length discrepancy

Figure 5.1 Congenital and functional leg length

Functional LLDs are those that occur as a result of alteration in lower-limb mechanics such as joint malalignment, muscle weakness, knee hyperextension, lumbar scoliosis and joint contracture. These problems can occur due to an abnormal movement in any of the three planes of the lower limb (Collebrusco *et al.*, 2020).

However, despite the theoretical difference in the definition of these two LLD types, they are not easily distinguishable in clinical practice. In fact, the use of non-functional assessment (e.g. radiography) is often unsuitable to determine the faulty lower-limb mechanics related to functional LLDs (Khamis and Carmeli, 2017).

Treatment controversy

There exists no doubt that a true and significant LLD can lead to functional compromise and other problems. When treating patients with LLD, however, appropriate care and some caution need to be exercised. Often, manual therapists have a tendency to apply different manipulative or mobilisation techniques even if the difference in leg length is marginal and causes no problems. Other manual therapeutic examination and treatment approaches (e.g. Derifield-Thompson) focus on the diagnosis and correction of upper cervical spine dysfunctions as these are thought to be manipulation-correctable causes of some forms of LLD (Shambaugh *et al.*, 1988).

Some even consider insignificant LLDs of 3–5 mm as clinically relevant and try to treat them, although they are not actually a problem to be corrected. Thus, before applying the therapy, an important question that needs to be asked is whether there will be any real benefit to the patient from its application or whether it will create an environment for patient harm. The therapist should consider the fact that limb-length inequality has been a subject of controversy for some time. In fact, to date, no consensus has been reached among clinical investigators and researchers regarding the acceptable range of LLD that requires treatment. There has also been a long debate about the long-term effects of LLD on function and the role it plays in different musculoskeletal disorders (Collebrusco *et al.*, 2020; Vogt *et al.*, 2020).

It is likely that the differences of opinion in existing medical literature are responsible for such eagerness among manual therapists to treat minute changes in LLDs. While some authors have suggested correcting LLDs of 3–12 mm even if the patient is asymptomatic (Gogia and Braatz, 1986; Gurney, 2002), others consider as much as 20–30 mm of LLDs to be clinically significant (Reid and Smith, 1984; Khamis and Carmeli, 2017). In terms of changes in gait, some authors reported no significant deviations in gait unless the discrepancy in leg length is considerably larger LLD (60 mm) (Gurney, 2002), while others have found abnormalities in gait with relatively small LLDs (20–30 mm) (Kaufman *et al.*, 1996; Bhave *et al.*, 1999; Gurney *et al.*, 2001). These wide spectrum disagreements in the current literature, however, can largely be attributed to the various measurement methods utilised in these studies and their poor validity and reliability in measuring LLD (Khamis and Carmeli, 2017). In fact, the most commonly used method (tape measure) of measuring LLD by manual therapists has been found to be highly inaccurate compared with radiography (Farahmand *et al.*, 2019). Studies have reported an estimated measuring error of ± 8.6 mm to ± 10.1 mm with this method (Woerman and Binder-Macleod, 1984; Friberg *et al.*, 1988).

Although there is little consensus about the magnitude of LLD that warrants corrective treatment, some authors have suggested a general outline to help in clinical decision making regarding what extent of LLD can be considered significant. Reid and Smith (1984) suggested three categories of LLD:

- Mild (0–30 mm) LLD – treatment may not be needed at all; if needed, treatment should be non-surgical.

- Moderate (30–60 mm) LLD – a case-to-case approach is needed; some cases may require surgical corrections.

- Severe (> 60 mm) LLD – surgical correction is needed.

A similar breakdown is also proposed by Moseley (1996), where no treatment is suggested for 0–20 mm of LLD, a shoe lift or shortening for 20–60 mm, lengthening for 60–200 mm, and prosthetic fitting for > 200 mm. In addition, it has been found that discrepancies of 5–25 mm are not functionally detrimental to marathon runners (Gross, 1983). The impact of LLD may also vary with the magnitude and frequency of impact activity. A more recent study investigating the impact of LLD on high school cross-country runners (Rauh, 2018) concluded that those with a greater than 1.5 cm LLD possess a greater likelihood of acquiring repetitive running injuries (RRI). Recently, after reviewing the available literature, Gordon and Davis (2019) concluded that there appeared to be a consensus that LLDs of > 20 mm could frequently be a problem. The authors, however, also suggested that LLDs as small as 5 mm are not negligible and have some evidence for long-term pathology.

Taken together, manual therapists need to make a sound clinical decision before deciding to treat individuals with LLD. They should consider each clinical problem of LLD on a case-to-case basis and take several factors into consideration, including the degree of LLD, the presence or absence of pain and/or restriction in function, whether there is a history of frequent back pain, existence of a marked inequality in the upper limbs and the likelihood of future musculoskeletal problems (Gurney, 2002; Vogt *et al.*, 2020). It is also important to differentiate correctly between anatomic LLD and functional LLD during the assessment (Collebrusco *et al.*, 2020). Even if the magnitude of LLD is the same, individuals with acquired LLDs can have more debilitating symptoms than those with congenital LLDs (Etnier and Landers, 1998). Thus, a correct assessment of LLDs is critically important to decide whether there is a need for manual therapy intervention.

Methods of measuring LLD

Up to now, imaging techniques such as radiography, computerised tomography (CT), magnetic resonance imaging (MRI) and 3D ultrasonography have been the most accurate and reliable methods to measure LLD. Of these, CT has shown to have better reproducibility and accuracy for measuring LLD than other imaging techniques (Sabharwal and Kumar, 2008). The use of radiography, however, is more common than other techniques owing to its comparatively lower cost. It is still considered the gold standard for accurate LLD measurement. In clinical practice, three types of radiographs are commonly utilised to measure LLD: orthoroentgenogram, scanogram and computerised digital radiograph. These radiographic techniques usually measure the distance between the proximal femur and the ankle using some landmarks (Gurney, 2002).

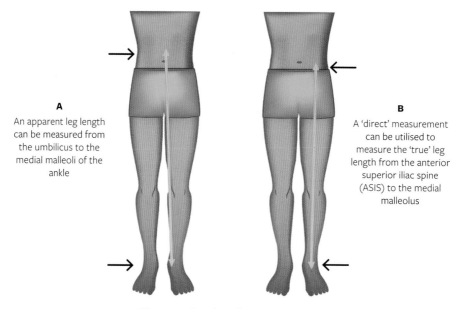

A
An apparent leg length can be measured from the umbilicus to the medial malleoli of the ankle

B
A 'direct' measurement can be utilised to measure the 'true' leg length from the anterior superior iliac spine (ASIS) to the medial malleolus

Figure 5.2 Leg-length measurements

The EOS® imaging system has also evolved to be a low-dose weight-bearing LLD assessment imaging modality particularly for children and scoliosis-related LLD (Escott *et al.* 2013).

There are, however, some major drawbacks to the use of these imaging techniques. They are not generalisable for all patients due to their high cost, complex method and time-consuming procedures. Some techniques such as radiography and CT also expose patients to radiation. Their use in the routine clinical setting is therefore impractical (Harvey *et al.*, 2010). Instead, manual therapists commonly use two alternative clinical methods to measure LLD: the direct method and the indirect method. These clinical methods are cheaper, easier and less time-consuming, but they have limited reliability and validity. Hence, it might be misleading to make a clinical decision about the need for intervention based on their results (Khamis and Carmeli, 2017; Farahmand *et al.*, 2019).

The direct method is performed with the patient lying in a supine position. It utilises a measuring tape to assess the distance between the anterior superior iliac spine (ASIS) and the medial or lateral malleolus. Although there is controversy regarding the accuracy of this method, some authors suggest that the average of two tape measurements between the above anatomical points seems to have good validity and reliability if used as a screening tool for measuring LLD (Jamaluddin *et al.*, 2011; Neelly *et al.*, 2013).

The indirect method, on the other hand, is done with the patient standing. In this method, lift blocks of defined height are placed below the short leg. The therapist gradually corrects the shortening using blocks until the pelvis is level. The leg-length difference is the total height of the blocks needed to level the pelvis (Petrone *et al.*, 2003). An advantage of this method over the direct method is that it incorporates functional factors such as hip, knee, foot and ankle position. However, a downside is that it could give false-positive results if the loading of the legs is asymmetrical while standing. Regarding the reliability and validity of this method, there are conflicting opinions in the literature as to whether it is superior or inferior to the direct method (Gurney, 2002; Khamis and Carmeli, 2017).

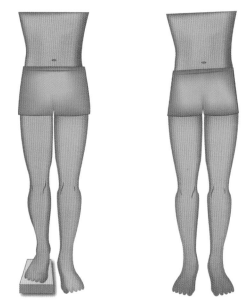

Measuring leg-length discrepancy using the block method
Level pelvis is achieved by equalisation with blocks of 4 cm in total height

Figure 5.3 Block method of measuring LLD

Taken together, because clinical methods have limited validity and reliability, we recommend that manual therapists should utilise imaging techniques to measure LLD if accuracy is critical to making a clinical decision regarding intervention.

References

Bhave, A., Paley, D. and Herzenberg, J.E. (1999) Improvement in gait parameters after lengthening for the treatment of limb-length discrepancy. *Journal of Bone and Joint Surgery 81*, 4, 529–534.

Bialosky, J.E., Bishop, M.D., George, S.Z. and Robinson, M.E. (2011) Placebo response to manual therapy: Something out of nothing? *Journal of Manual and Manipulative Therapy 19*, 1, 11–19.

Boyling, J.D. and Jull, G.A. (eds) (2004) *Grieve's Modern Manual Therapy*. Churchill Livingstone.

Brady, R.J., Dean, J.B., Skinner, T.M. and Gross, M.T. (2003) Limb length inequality: Clinical implications for assessment and intervention. *Journal of Orthopaedic and Sports Physical Therapy 33*, 5, 221–234.

Cochran, T.M., Mu, K., Lohman, H. and Scheirton, L.S. (2009) Physical therapists' perspectives on practice errors in geriatric, neurologic, or orthopedic clinical settings. *Physiotherapy Theory and Practice 25*, 1, 1–13.

Collebrusco, L., Censi, G. and Casoli, P. (2020) The question of short lower limb and long lower in manual therapy: An overview. *Open Journal of Therapy and Rehabilitation 8*, 4, 143–152.

Cook, C. (2011) *Orthopedic Manual Therapy*. Prentice Hall.

Escott, B.G., Ravi, B., Weathermon, A.C., Acharya, J. *et al.* (2013) EOS low-dose radiography: A reliable and accurate upright assessment of lower-limb lengths. *Journal of Bone and Joint Surgery 95*, 23, e1831–e1837.

Etnier, J.L. and Landers, D.M. (1998) Motor performance and motor learning as a function of age and fitness. *Research Quarterly for Exercise and Sport 69*, 2, 136–146.

Farahmand, B., Takamjani, E.E., Yazdi, H.R., Saeedi, H., Kamali, M. and Cham, M.B. (2019) A systematic review on the validity and reliability of tape measurement method in leg length discrepancy. *Medical Journal of the Islamic Republic of Iran 33*, 46.

Friberg, O., Nurminen, M., Korhonen, K., Soininen, E. and Mänttäri, T. (1988) Accuracy and precision of clinical estimation of leg length inequality and lumbar scoliosis: Comparison of clinical and radiological measurements. *International Disability Studies 10*, 2, 49–53.

Gogia, P.P. and Braatz, J.H. (1986) Validity and reliability of leg length measurements. *Journal of Orthopaedic and Sports Physical Therapy 8*, 4, 185–188.

Gordon, J.E. and Davis, L.E. (2019) Leg length discrepancy: The natural history (and what do we really know). *Journal of Pediatric Orthopaedics 39*, S10–S13.

Gross, R.H. (1983) Leg length discrepancy in marathon runners. *The American Journal of Sports Medicine 11*, 3, 121–124.

Guichet, J.M., Spivak, J.M., Trouilloud, P. and Grammont, P.M. (1991) Lower limb-length discrepancy: An epidemiologic study. *Clinical Orthopaedics and Related Research 1991*, 272, 235–241.

Gurney, B. (2002) Leg length discrepancy. *Gait and Posture 15*, 2, 195–206.

Gurney, B., Mermier, C., Robergs, R., Gibson, A. and Rivero, D. (2001) Effects of limb-length discrepancy on gait economy and lower-extremity muscle activity in older adults. *Journal of Bone and Joint Surgery 83*, 6, 907–915.

Harvey, W.F., Yang, M., Cooke, T.D., Segal, N.A. *et al.* (2010) Association of leg-length inequality with knee osteoarthritis: A cohort study. *Annals of Internal Medicine 152*, 5, 287–295.

Hasler, C.C. (2000) Leg length inequality: Indications for treatment and importance of shortening procedures. *Der Orthopade 29*, 9, 766–774.

Hellsing, A.L. (1988) Leg length inequality: A prospective study of young men during their military service. *Upsala Journal of Medical Sciences 93*, 3, 245–253.

Jamaluddin, S., Sulaiman, A.R., Kamarul Imran, M., Juhara, H., Ezane, M.A. and Nordin, S. (2011) Reliability and accuracy of the tape measurement method with a nearest reading of 5 mm in the assessment of leg length discrepancy. *Singapore Medical Journal 52*, 9, 681–684.

Kaufman, K.R., Miller, L.S. and Sutherland, D.H. (1996) Gait asymmetry in patients with limb-length inequality. *Journal of Pediatric Orthopaedics 16*, 2, 144–150.

Khamis, S. and Carmeli, E. (2017) A new concept for measuring leg length discrepancy. *Journal of Orthopaedics 14*, 2, 276–280.

Knutson, G.A. (2005) Anatomic and functional leg-length inequality: A review and recommendation for clinical decision-making. Part I, anatomic leg-length inequality: Prevalence, magnitude, effects and clinical significance. *Chiropractic and Osteopathy 13*, 1, 1–10.

Lederman, E. (2005) *The Science and Practice of Manual Therapy*, 2nd edn. Elsevier Health Sciences.

Moseley, C.F. (1996) Leg Length Discrepancy and Angular Deformity of the Lower Limbs. In R.T. Morrissy and S.L. Weinstein (eds) *Lovell and Winter's Pediatric Orthopedics*, 4th edn. Lippincott-Raven.

Neely, K., Wallmann, H.W. and Backus, C.J. (2013) Validity of measuring leg length with a tape measure compared to a computed tomography scan. *Physiotherapy Theory and Practice 29*, 6, 487–492.

Petrone, M.R., Guinn, J., Reddin, A., Sutlive, T.G., Flynn, T.W. and Garber, M.P. (2003) The accuracy of the palpation meter (PALM) for measuring pelvic crest height difference and leg length discrepancy. *Journal of Orthopaedic and Sports Physical Therapy 33*, 6, 319–325.

Rauh, M.J. (2018) Leg-length inequality and running-related injury among high school runners. *International Journal of Sports Physical Therapy 13*, 4, 643–651.

Reid, D.C. and Smith, B. (1984) Leg length inequality: A review of etiology and management. *Physiotherapy Canada 36*, 4, 177–182.

Sabharwal, S. and Kumar, A. (2008) Methods for assessing leg length discrepancy. *Clinical Orthopaedics and Related Research 466*, 12, 2910–2922.

Shambaugh, P., Sclafani, L. and Fanselow, D. (1988) Reliability of the Derifield-Thompson test for leg length inequality, and use of the test to demonstrate cervical adjusting efficacy. *Journal of Manipulative and Physiological Therapeutics 11*, 5, 396–399.

Vogt, B., Gosheger, G., Wirth, T., Horn, J. and Rödl, R. (2020) Leg length discrepancy – treatment indications and strategies. *Deutsches Ärzteblatt International 117*, 24, 405–411.

Woerman, A.L. and Binder-Macleod, S.A. (1984) Leg length discrepancy assessment: Accuracy and precision in five clinical methods of evaluation. *Journal of Orthopaedic and Sports Physical Therapy 5*, 5, 230–239.

Chapter 6

Patient Referral – When to Stop

DR KUMAR KUNASINGAM

You will never be criticised for being cautious, you will only be criticised for being cavalier.

This statement highlights the need to always ensure that we put the patient first, acknowledge our limitations and understand when treatment should stop and when a referral to other healthcare practitioners may be appropriate.

As an orthopaedic surgeon, I believe teamwork is vital. The communication between manual therapist, doctor and potential surgical referral and then back to manual therapy post-operation needs to be open and honest, clear and effective, and patient-centred not self-centred. This chapter gives a brief look at when to consider stopping treatment and when to consider X-ray, MRI or medical referral for foot and ankle conditions.

Manual therapists are increasingly becoming first-contact providers in the healthcare system. Many healthcare networks and even some hospitals now utilise manual therapists as the first point of care to examine or triage patients with musculoskeletal disorders or injuries (Keil *et al.*, 2019). In several developed countries, it has also become an established practice model to allow imaging referral privileges to manual therapists. Although the current evidence is limited in support of direct access to manual therapy or similar modalities, the available evidence suggests that having manual therapists in such roles may reduce the overall cost of care, the number of surgeries performed, the wait time for imaging studies and delays in receiving manual therapy treatment (Jette *et al.*, 2006; Keil *et al.*, 2019; Keil *et al.*, 2021).

The fundamental challenge for manual therapists, however, is to make correct clinical decisions regarding whether to treat or refer a patient. In general, timely referral for specialist care by manual therapists primarily depends on their ability to screen for differential diagnostic pathologies (Budtz *et al.*, 2021). This involves utilising sound clinical reasoning, which is a complex reflective process where a therapist develops and tests differential diagnostic hypotheses based on the patient's medical history, physical examination findings and response to treatment. This also includes having sound knowledge of the red flags, precautions and contraindications for manual therapy treatment (Huhn *et al.*, 2019; Ziebart and MacDermid, 2019).

Clinical practice guidelines and textbooks on manual therapy have long suggested screening for serious pathologies at each patient encounter as part of the normal assessment process. These resources also summarise clinical red flags and other signs that need immediate medical attention (Boissonnault and Ross, 2012). To date, however, little research has been carried out to understand the evaluative and diagnostic processes that manual therapists utilise for clinical decision making during patient referral. In addition, little is yet known regarding their ability and confidence in screening for serious medical conditions (Boyles *et al.*, 2011; Keil *et al.*, 2019).

Studies published up to now, however, have consistently reported poor management decisions by manual therapists in critical medical categories (Budtz *et al.*, 2021). The most likely reason for this is the fact that, in the past, their training and education were primarily focused on physical examination, not medical diagnosis (Jette *et al.*, 2006). This has brought changes in the entry-level educational curricula of manual therapy; most programmes now include imaging content in their curricula (Boissonnault *et al.*, 2014; Keil *et al.*, 2021). Still, two of the major concerns are appropriateness and overuse of diagnostic imaging by manual therapists (Boyles *et al.*, 2011). Two recent studies, however, have reported favourable results supporting imaging referral by manual therapists and found consistency with established criteria in both overall use rate and imaging referrals (Crowell *et al.*, 2016; Keil *et al.*, 2019). Furthermore, the American Physical Therapy Association (APTA) has recently published an Imaging Education Manual for the integration of imaging content into the doctor of manual therapy educational program (APTA, 2015).

This chapter describes the evaluative processes related to imaging referral by manual therapists for foot and ankle conditions. We also discuss the clinical scenario for which a referral to a general physician or orthopaedic surgeon should be indicated.

Patient referral for diagnostic imaging: how to proceed

Manual therapists should carefully consider the following elements before deciding to utilise diagnostic imaging:

- patient history

- clinical examination findings

- response to conservative management

- other emerging clinical factors.

The APTA Imaging Education Manual (APTA, 2015) and the imaging practice guidelines for chiropractors (Bussières *et al.*, 2007a, 2007b) recommend following the Ottawa ankle and foot rules for specific imaging decision guidance (see below). This should be taken into consideration during the decision-making process. Another important component that is often underrepresented in the literature is the collaboration between manual therapists and radiologists. However, the role of effective communication in the direct imaging referral process is significant. This is because the quality of information exchange with the radiologist can help to determine the most appropriate imaging procedure and subsequently improve patient management decisions (European Society of Radiology, 2013).

Once a manual therapist deems diagnostic imaging necessary, the next stage is to create a timely and appropriate referral. It is of critical importance for manual therapists to provide sufficient clinical information to the radiologist as part of the referral. Often, the only salient information provided in the referral is the clinical notes that the radiologist receives other than the image itself. If the radiologist has the necessary information regarding the clinical problem for which the imaging procedure is ordered, this will yield more relevant clinical information within the report (Pitman, 2017; Keil *et al.*, 2021). Table 6.1 highlights the key information that needs to be included in a routine imaging referral.

Table 6.1 Clinical information that should be included
in a manual therapy imaging referral

Key elements	Details that must be provided
Patient	Name and contact information (e.g. postal address, phone number, email)
Referring manual therapist	Name and contact information (e.g. postal address, phone and fax number, email)
Clinical summary	This should briefly detail the need for imaging, including the following information: • Mechanism of injury • Anatomic location of injury, pain or tenderness • Results of clinical tests (clearly state whether the suspected pathology is positive, negative or inconclusive) • Neurovascular status (if neurological conditions such as Morton's neuroma or nerve entrapment are suspected) • Results of previous imaging studies (if available)
Hypothesised clinical diagnosis	Clearly state the suspected condition or the diagnosed pathology that needs further study
Imaging order	Clearly state the imaging procedure that needs to be performed
Urgency of report	Clearly state whether the report is needed more urgently than the usual reporting timeline

Adapted from Keil et al. (2021)

The Ottawa ankle and foot rules

The Ottawa ankle and foot rules are a set of clinical decision-making directives for clinicians to determine the need for radiographic imaging in ankle and foot injuries. This screening tool, finalised in 1995, was developed to eliminate unnecessary imaging requests, avoid undue exposure to radiation, increase the throughput in the emergency department and reduce the cost of care (Herman, 2021).

The Ottawa rules have remained the gold standard of care for clinical decision making in ankle and foot injuries that require radiographic imaging. The sensitivity of this instrument is almost 100% while the specificity is fairly modest (about 30%) (Barelds *et al.*, 2017; Beckenkamp *et al.*, 2017). The instrument's proper application has been reported to reduce the need for unnecessary radiographs by 30–40% (Bachmann *et al.*, 2003). Other protocols and techniques have been developed over the years that equal the Ottawa tool; however, it surpasses all of them in terms of its reliability, simplicity and reproducibility (Herman, 2021).

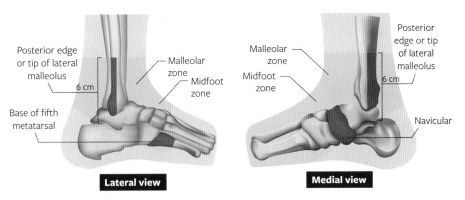

Figure 6.1 The Ottawa ankle and foot rules

Rules for ankle radiographs

Clinicians should request an ankle radiograph only if the patient complains of any pain in the malleolar zone and presents with any one of the following:

- bone tenderness at the posterior edge of the fibula or tip of the lateral malleolus (the lower 6 cm of the fibula)

- bone tenderness at the posterior edge of the tibia or tip of the medial malleolus (the lower 6 cm of the tibia)

- inability to bear weight or walk for at least four steps on the affected limb both immediately after the injury and in the casualty department.

Rules for foot radiographs

Clinicians should request foot radiographs only if the patient complains of any pain in the midfoot zone and presents with either of the following:

- point tenderness at the fifth metatarsal base or the navicular bone

- inability to bear weight or walk for at least four steps on the affected limb both immediately after the injury and in the casualty department.

Exceptions

The Ottawa ankle and foot rules do not apply to certain patient groups. These include:

- age < 5 years old

- pregnant women

- patients with ankle or foot injury more than ten days old

- patients who are unable to follow the test (e.g. intoxicated or uncooperative individuals)

- patients with diminished sensation in their lower limbs

- patients with painful injuries in other regions of the body

- patients in whom palpation is not possible in the malleolar zone due to gross swelling.

In the above cases, the clinical reasoning of the therapist should prevail over the Ottawa rules.

Recommendations for diagnostic imaging

Radiography

The APTA Imaging Education Manual (APTA, 2015) and the chiropractic practice guidelines for diagnostic imaging (Bussières *et al.*, 2007a) recommend ordering radiographic imaging if any one of the following ankle and foot conditions is suspected or needs further study:

- chronic ankle or foot pain

- stress fracture

- foot or ankle joint instability

- penetrating trauma

- acute toe injury

- osteonecrosis

- complex regional pain syndrome

- joint degeneration

- impingement syndromes (anterolateral, anterior, anteromedial and posterior)

- Morton's neuroma

- osteomyelitis in diabetic foot.

Bussières *et al.* (2007a) suggested a list of foot and ankle conditions in which radiography is not routinely indicated. These include:

- acute ankle and foot injury with negative findings on the Ottawa rules
- peroneal tendinosis
- lateral premalleolar bursitis
- tarsal tunnel syndrome
- plantar fasciitis and calcaneal enthesophyte (spur)
- sinus tarsi syndrome
- midfoot pain (non-traumatic)
- forefoot pain
- hindfoot-heel pain
- acquired flat foot with posterior tibial tendon dysfunction/rupture
- metatarsal bursitis
- navicular tuberosity pain and tenderness
- hallux rigidus and hallux valgus (first MTP joint)
- sesamoiditis.

Advanced imaging

In certain ankle and foot conditions, advanced imaging (e.g. magnetic resonance imaging, computed tomography, ultrasound or scintigraphy) and/or orthopaedic referral are recommended. Table 6.2 highlights the foot and ankle pathologies that require special investigation.

Table 6.2 Recommendation for special investigations
in various ankle and foot conditions

Clinical presentation	Recommendation	Comments
Acute ankle or foot fracture (positive findings on the Ottawa tool)	Special investigations and orthopaedic referral are recommended	MRI or CT should be performed if there is significant pain and disability and X-ray findings are negative Fluoroscopy or US under anaesthesia may be performed if ankle instability is suspected Scintigraphy may be indicated if there are persisting symptoms indicative of stress fracture
Stress fracture (fatigue or insufficiency)	Special investigations and orthopaedic referral are recommended if X-ray findings are inconclusive	MRI or scintigraphy may be indicated to optimally visualise the affected lesion and its surrounding structures
Impingement syndromes (anterolateral, anterior, anteromedial or posterior)	Special investigations and orthopaedic referral are warranted if there are positive X-ray findings and no improvements after four weeks of conservative care	Contrast-enhanced, three-dimensional, fat-suppressed, T1 or T2 weighted MRI may be performed for optimal visualisation (Al-Riyami et al., 2017)
Peroneal tendinosis	Radiographic imaging and special investigations are indicated if there is no improvement after four weeks of conservative care or the patient shows symptoms of inflammatory arthritis	MRI or US may be indicated if popping or clicking occurs with foot eversion
Posterior tibial tendon dysfunction	Radiographic imaging is indicated if there is no improvement after four weeks of conservative care or the patient shows symptoms of inflammatory arthritis Special investigations are indicated if radiography is positive or no improvement is seen with conservative care	MRI and high-resolution US may be used to exclude medial ankle/foot pain and for the accurate detection of the condition (Arnoldner et al., 2015)
Lateral premalleolar bursitis	Special investigations are indicated if there is no improvement after four weeks of conservative care	US may be indicated to optimally visualise the affected lesion and its surrounding vascularity

Tarsal tunnel syndrome	Special investigations and orthopaedic referral are recommended	MRI or US is indicated for visualisation of the posterior tibial nerve and other soft tissue CT may be performed to detect bony abnormalities Consider orthopaedic referral if there is persistent pain and disability and the conservative therapy fails
Sinus tarsi syndrome	Special investigations are indicated if no improvement is seen after four weeks of conservative care	MRI provides the best imaging to detect subtle unilateral deformities and see changes within the structure of the sinus tarsi (Helgeson, 2009)
Hindfoot-heel pain	Special investigations and orthopaedic referral are indicated if no improvement is seen after four weeks of conservative care	X-ray may be indicated for the differential diagnosis of the calcaneus and tarsal coalition trauma MRI may be useful
Midfoot pain (non-traumatic)	Radiographic imaging is indicated if there is no improvement after four weeks of conservative care or the patient shows symptoms of inflammatory arthritis Special investigations are indicated if radiography is positive or no improvement is seen with conservative care	CT or MRI is indicated for the investigation of suspected or further study of proven disease, or if there are negative/equivocal X-ray findings
Forefoot pain	Radiographic imaging is indicated if there is no improvement after four weeks of conservative care or the pain is suspected to be of inflammatory or infectious aetiology Special investigations are indicated if no improvement is seen with four weeks of conservative care	MRI should be indicated for the differential diagnosis of various forefoot conditions such as hallux valgus, stress fracture, sesamoiditis or metatarsal bursitis
Navicular tuberosity pain and tenderness	Radiographic imaging is indicated if there is no improvement after four weeks of conservative care Special investigations are indicated if no improvement is seen with four weeks of conservative care	MRI and/or scintigraphy may be used for differential diagnosis and to confirm the location of pain
Complex regional pain syndrome	Special investigations and orthopaedic referral are recommended	Scintigraphy should be indicated if X-ray findings are not diagnostic (Wertli et al., 2017). MRI may be useful for better visualisation of bones, joint processes and soft-tissue structures

Clinical presentation	Recommendation	Comments
Plantar fasciitis and calcaneal enthesophyte (spur)	Special investigations and orthopaedic referral are recommended (but not critical)	X-ray may be indicated for young athletes Doppler/power US may be indicated for initial assessment. MRI and scintigraphy may be used to visualise inflammatory changes (Draghi et al., 2017)
Osteonecrosis (avascular necrosis)	Special investigations and orthopaedic referral are warranted if there are positive X-ray findings	MRI should be indicated to assess the changes in bone marrow during the early stages
Sesamoiditis	Radiographic imaging is indicated if there is no improvement after four weeks of conservative care Special investigations are indicated for differential diagnosis	MRI may be indicated to exclude turf toe

CT: computed tomography; MRI: magnetic resonance imaging; US: ultrasound.

Adapted from Bussières et al. (2007a, 2007b); APTA (2015)

Box 6.1 Clinical scenarios that need urgent medical care or referral to a specialist after positive imaging findings

- Acute ankle or foot fracture (positive on the Ottawa rules)

- Peripheral neuropathy

- Complete muscle tear or disruption

- Dislocations of the ankle and foot joints

- Septic arthritis

- Cancer with constitutional symptoms

- Infection or neoplasm

- Vascular conditions (e.g. chronic venous insufficiency, deep vein thrombosis, post-thrombotic syndrome or peripheral artery disease)

Adapted from Keil et al. (2021)

References

Al-Riyami, A.M., Tan, H.K. and Peh, W.C. (2017) Imaging of ankle impingement syndromes. *Canadian Association of Radiologists Journal 68*, 4, 431–437.

American Physical Therapy Association (2015) *Imaging Education Manual for Doctor of Physical Therapy Professional Degree Programs*, www.orthopt.org/uploads/content_files/ISIG/IMAGING_EDUCATION_MANUAL_FINAL_4.15.15..pdf

Arnoldner, M.A., Gruber, M., Syré, S., Kristen, K.H. *et al.* (2015) Imaging of posterior tibial tendon dysfunction: Comparison of high-resolution ultrasound and 3 T MRI. *European Journal of Radiology 84*, 9, 1777–1781.

Bachmann, L.M., Kolb, E., Koller, M.T., Steurer, J. and ter Riet, G. (2003) Accuracy of Ottawa ankle rules to exclude fractures of the ankle and mid-foot: Systematic review. *BMJ 326*, 7386, 417.

Barelds, I., Krijnen, W.P., van de Leur, J.P., van der Schans, C.P. and Goddard, R.J. (2017) Diagnostic accuracy of clinical decision rules to exclude fractures in acute ankle injuries: Systematic review and meta-analysis. *The Journal of Emergency Medicine 53*, 3, 353–368.

Beckenkamp, P.R., Lin, C.W.C., Macaskill, P., Michaleff, Z.A., Maher, C.G. and Moseley, A.M. (2017) Diagnostic accuracy of the Ottawa Ankle and Midfoot Rules: A systematic review with meta-analysis. *British Journal of Sports Medicine 51*, 6, 504–510.

Boissonnault, W.G. and Ross, M.D. (2012) Physical therapists referring patients to physicians: A review of case reports and series. *Journal of Orthopedic and Sports Physical Therapy 42*, 5, 446–454.

Boissonnault, W.G., White, D.M., Carney, S., Malin, B. and Smith, W. (2014) Diagnostic and procedural imaging curricula in physical therapist professional degree programs. *Journal of Orthopedic and Sports Physical Therapy 44*, 8, 579–586.

Boyles, R.E., Gorman, I., Pinto, D. and Ross, M.D. (2011) Physical therapist practice and the role of diagnostic imaging. *Journal of Orthopedic and Sports Physical Therapy 41*, 11, 829–837.

Budtz, C.R., Rønn-Smidt, H., Thomsen, J.N.L., Hansen, R.P. and Christiansen, D.H. (2021) Primary care physiotherapists ability to make correct management decision – is there room for improvement? A mixed method study. *BMC Family Practice 22*, 1, 1–10.

Bussières, A.E., Peterson, C. and Taylor, J.A. (2007a) Diagnostic imaging practice guidelines for musculoskeletal complaints in adults – an evidence-based approach: Introduction. *Journal of Manipulative and Physiological Therapeutics 30*, 9, 617–683.

Bussières, A.E., Taylor, J.A. and Peterson, C. (2007b) Diagnostic imaging practice guidelines for musculoskeletal complaints in adults – an evidence-based approach: Part 1: Lower extremity disorders. *Journal of Manipulative and Physiological Therapeutics 30*, 9, 684–717.

Crowell, M.S., Dedekam, E.A., Johnson, M.R., Dembowski, S.C., Westrick, R.B. and Goss, D.L. (2016) Diagnostic imaging in a direct-access sports physical therapy clinic: A 2-year retrospective practice analysis. *International Journal of Sports Physical Therapy 11*, 5, 708–717.

Draghi, F., Gitto, S., Bortolotto, C., Draghi, A.G. and Belometti, G.O. (2017) Imaging of plantar fascia disorders: Findings on plain radiography, ultrasound and magnetic resonance imaging. *Insights into Imaging 8*, 1, 69–78.

European Society of Radiology (ESR) (2013) ESR communication guidelines for radiologists. *Insights into Imaging 4*, 143–146.

Helgeson, K. (2009) Examination and intervention for sinus tarsi syndrome. *North American Journal of Sports Physical Therapy: NAJSPT 4*, 1, 29–37.

Herman, L. (2021) A 20-year perspective on the Ottawa Ankle Rules: Are we still on solid footing? *Journal of the American Academy of Physician Assistants 34*, 7, 15–20.

Huhn, K., Gilliland, S.J., Black, L.L., Wainwright, S.F. and Christensen, N. (2019) Clinical reasoning in physical therapy: A concept analysis. *Physical Therapy 99*, 4, 440–456.

Jette, D.U., Ardleigh, K., Chandler, K. and McShea, L. (2006) Decision-making ability of physical therapists: Physical therapy intervention or medical referral. *Physical Therapy 86*, 12, 1619–1629.

Keil, A.P., Baranyi, B., Mehta, S. and Maurer, A. (2019) Ordering of diagnostic imaging by physical therapists: A 5-year retrospective practice analysis. *Physical Therapy 99*, 8, 1020–1026.

Keil, A.P., Hazle, C., Maurer, A., Kittleson, C. *et al.* (2021) Referral for imaging in physical therapist practice: Key recommendations for successful implementation. *Physical Therapy 101*, 3, pzab013.

Pitman, A.G. (2017) Quality of referral: What information should be included in a request for diagnostic imaging when a patient is referred to a clinical radiologist? *Journal of Medical Imaging and Radiation Oncology 61*, 3, 299–303.

Wertli, M.M., Brunner, F., Steurer, J. and Held, U. (2017) Usefulness of bone scintigraphy for the diagnosis of Complex Regional Pain Syndrome 1: A systematic review and Bayesian meta-analysis. *PLOS ONE 12*, 3, e0173688.

Ziebart, C. and MacDermid, J.C. (2019) Reflective practice in physical therapy: A scoping review. *Physical Therapy 99*, 8, 1056–1068.

Chapter 7

Use of Orthotics in Foot and Ankle Disorders

Ankle and foot orthoses, braces or splints are external devices commonly used to help improve or support the normal functioning of the foot and/or ankle. The primary goals for using these devices are to enable the patient to offload pressure from specific foot or ankle regions, halt the further progression of a foot or ankle pathology and maintain a neutral or near neutral ankle joint alignment through the various stages of gait. Orthopaedic physicians and physical therapy practitioners frequently prescribe these devices to various patient groups, in particular those with a foot or ankle condition that compromises sensation/proprioception, normal walking ability, skin integrity and muscle, joint or motor function. Examples of these groups include children with congenital disorders (e.g. cerebral palsy), patients with systemic disorders affecting foot or ankle function (e.g. osteoarthritis, gout, diabetes), and those with overuse conditions (e.g. plantar fasciitis, Achilles tendinopathy, posterior tibial tendon dysfunction) (Janisse and Janisse, 2008; Elattar *et al.*, 2018).

Orthotic professionals have a long-held notion that orthotic devices, particularly foot orthoses, can correct mechanical abnormalities. The reason behind this conviction, however, is primarily visual, as, in most cases, there may be some apparent mechanical corrections after using the devices such as a perceived 'over-pronated foot' correction. Nevertheless, this belief is not supported by well-established evidence (Harlaar *et al.*, 2010). Recent findings suggest that internal joint kinetics at the foot and ankle are more important for achieving therapeutic benefit. Moreover, the current evidence neither discards nor endorses the use of orthotics for therapeutic benefits or for promoting walking ability (Choo and Chang, 2021). In fact, the level of evidence presented in the current body of literature is largely of low quality, and the number of high-quality studies, especially randomised clinical trials, is still scarce (Landorf and Keenan, 2000; Ridgewell *et al.*, 2010; Aboutorabi *et al.*, 2017).

There is also a scarcity of prescription guidelines for the orthotic treatment of foot and ankle disorders. A major reason for this is the absence of conclusive evidence supporting the use of orthotic devices. Although several consensus reports have been published in recent years (Condie, 2004; Hijmans and Geertzen, 2006; Jarrett and Marcus, 2006; Fisk *et al.*, 2016), these reports are still inconclusive in many ways, particularly how and when a foot or ankle pathology should be supported or counteracted by orthotic devices and which device is more appropriate for a specific condition. There is also a lack of recommendation grades in these reports.

The lack of clarity in prescription guidelines is reflected in clinical practice as well, which can be seen with respect to both treatment indication and device type and material selection (Harlaar *et al.*, 2010). In fact, orthotic prescriptions may differ substantially between therapists (Menz *et al.*, 2017), and some therapists have a tendency to prescribe orthotics to almost every patient they encounter, even if they may not need them. This ultimately causes more harm to the patients instead of resolving their problems. This chapter, therefore, provides a general overview of the use of orthotics in foot and ankle conditions. We will also discuss how and when these devices should be used and when it is best to avoid them.

Ankle and foot orthoses

Ankle and foot orthoses are primarily used to achieve the following objectives (Elattar *et al.*, 2018):

- shock absorption and shock attenuation

- cushioning areas of tenderness

- offloading abnormally high plantar pressure through dissipation of weight-bearing pressures across the plantar surface

- supporting and protecting healed fracture sites (total-contact concept)

- minimising high shear forces

- correcting or stabilising flexible deformities

- limiting or controlling motion of painful joints

- accommodating rigid or fixed deformities.

Ankle and foot orthoses are readily available in two types: custom-made devices and prefabricated off-the-shelf devices. Both are made from a variety of materials that vary in density, thickness, cushioning capacity, shock absorption and flexibility (Janisse and Janisse, 2008).

Custom-made orthoses

Custom foot orthoses are usually made from a plaster cast, model or 3D scan of the patient's foot. Most often, commercial laboratories manufacture these devices following specifications requested by podiatrists. Custom orthoses have the advantage of more intimately fitting than prefabricated devices. They can be modified based on the patient-specific design features, which ultimately are assumed to provide more therapeutic benefits and patient comfort. A custom device is often prescribed for patients with a considerable foot or ankle deformity, loss of sensation/proprioception and a history of ulcers and/or arthropathy (Menz *et al.*, 2017; Fox and Lovegreen, 2019).

Custom foot orthoses can be divided into three types: accommodative orthoses, rigid orthoses and semi-rigid orthoses.

Accommodative foot orthoses

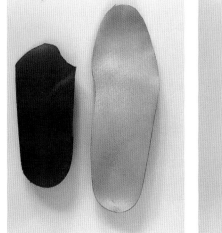
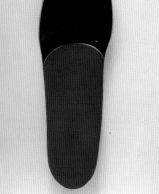

Figure 7.1 Orthotics 1　　　*Figure 7.2 Orthotics 2*

Accommodative orthotics are softer by design. They are made of less durable materials and thus require periodic follow-up, repair and replacement. These orthoses are primarily meant to cushion, pad and protect a painful or injured area of the foot. They can help attenuate the load of standing and walking, decrease friction shear forces across the sole and dissipate weight-bearing pressures away from injured areas (Janisse and Janisse, 2008).

Indications: Diabetic foot ulcers, small or minor deformities, painful calluses on the sole, aching heels and other uncomfortable conditions.

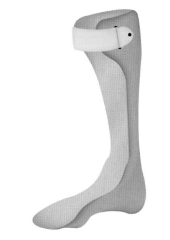

Figure 7.3 Moulded ankle and foot orthosis

Rigid foot orthoses

Rigid foot orthoses are usually made of durable materials such as thermo-plastics or carbon fibre composites. They provide excellent arch support for flexible deformities and offer an improvement in gait kinematics for those with ankle–foot instability. Rigid orthoses, however, are not easily adjustable and cannot be modified to accommodate plantar foot prominences. These orthoses are also not suitable for patients with peripheral neuropathy, as they are quite firm and less cushiony by design, and offer only minimal shock absorption and attenuation (Delafontaine *et al.*, 2017; Elattar *et al.*, 2018).

Indications: Severe ankle instability, drop foot, osteoarthritis and Charcot arthropathy.

Semi-rigid foot orthoses

Semi-rigid orthoses are a combination of both accommodative and rigid orthoses. They are usually made up of a firm supportive (base) layer with a soft, less dense top layer. The base offers support and control for flexible deformities and redistribution of weight-bearing pressures, while the soft layer provides cushioning and protection. Advantages of these orthoses include greater longevity than accommodative devices and easy adjustment and modifications, even for minor foot changes (Gross *et al.*, 2002; Elattar *et al.*, 2018).

Indications: Neuropathic foot pain, plantar fasciitis, diabetic foot ulcers, minor to major foot deformities, bony prominences associated with arthritis or Charcot arthropathy and other painful foot conditions.

Off-the-shelf orthoses

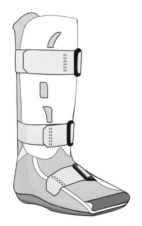

Figure 7.4 Off-the-shelf cam boot

Prefabricated, off-the-shelf orthoses are often indicated for minor foot problems, particularly in patients with neuropathy, ulcers or no deformity. The potential advantages of these devices include cheaper price, immediate availability and time conservation. Instead of waiting for weeks to have a custom-moulded device, the patient can have the prefabricated orthosis at the chairside just after the diagnosis and start wearing it in their own shoes immediately. However, compared with custom devices, these orthoses cannot intimately fit into shoes, have less longevity and are not easily adjustable. They are also not suitable for patients with sensory limitations or a history of ulcerations (Cameron-Fiddes and Santos, 2013; Elattar *et al.*, 2018; Fox and Lovegreen, 2019).

Indications: Plantar heel pain, diabetic foot ulcers, painful calluses on the sole and other minor foot conditions.

Prescribing foot orthoses

Prescribing the best possible orthosis for a patient is not a simple task. Physical therapists or similar professionals without expertise in orthotics should avoid prescribing these devices. This is because successful orthotic prescriptions require a thorough understanding of the lower-limb biomechanics. Therapists should be able to pinpoint areas of high pressure, determine limitations in range of motion and select the most appropriate orthosis according to the patient's condition (Janisse and Janisse, 2008; Elattar *et al.*, 2018). If possible, they should also involve an orthotist as part of the prescription process to ensure that the proper moulding technique and best materials and components are used.

Therapists should carefully consider the following aspects while selecting the type and design of the orthoses (Jarrett and Marcus, 2006):

- patient's medical history
- patient's beliefs
- body weight
- current footwear size and width
- mobility status
- activity level
- previous orthotic use
- systemic diseases
- muscle strength of the affected limb
- joint stability and range of motion
- gait pattern.

In addition, therapists should give special consideration to the time frame, which will depend on the condition as the patient may overuse or become dependent on their orthoses over time. In most foot or ankle conditions, orthoses should be used only in the short term. However, some specific conditions such as tibialis posterior dysfunction require the patient to use foot orthoses for their lifetime (Willy *et al.*, 2019). There is also a common belief that the use of orthoses can lead to weakening of foot muscles, although this is not supported by well-established evidence (Jung *et al.*, 2011; Protopapas and Perry, 2020). Nevertheless, if the therapist prescribes the orthosis properly, considering the individual patient's condition and needs, it can be a useful adjunct in combination with other interventions.

Clinical uses of orthoses in specific foot and ankle disorders

Orthotics are widely used as an adjunctive tool in the treatment of various ankle and foot conditions. Their usage varies from simple pain or discomfort relief to complete immobilisation. Table 7.1 summarises the most commonly used prefabricated and custom orthotics in different foot conditions.

Table 7.1 Clinical usage of orthotics in common foot and ankle conditions

Ankle/foot condition	Prescription orthotics
Plantar fasciitis	Both custom-made and off-the-shelf orthoses have been found to be equally effective for functional improvement in plantar heel pain (Tran and Spry, 2019)
	Both accommodative and semi-rigid orthoses can be useful
	Most commonly prescribed orthotics: prefabricated insoles, viscoelastic heel pads and night splints
	Duration of use: two weeks to 12 months (depending on the individual patient's condition)
Posterior tibial tendon dysfunction	Professionally prescribed, custom-moulded foot orthoses are useful for elderly, sedentary patients or those at high risk for surgery
	The selection of orthoses mainly depends on the type of deformity
	Complete restoration may be achieved for flexible deformity (stage II) with a custom orthosis
	In cases with rigid uncorrectable deformity (stage III), the brace is moulded to prevent the foot from collapsing into malalignment
	Most commonly prescribed orthotics: semi-rigid orthosis with arch support, rigid custom orthosis (Arizona brace)
	Duration of use: extended period or lifetime
Achilles tendinopathy	The use of semi-rigid custom insoles, heel lifts and night splints have been found to be helpful in patients' Achilles tendinopathy
	Most commonly prescribed orthotics: Arizona brace, AirHeel brace, heel lift, night splint
	Duration of use: two weeks to 12 months (depending on the individual patient's condition)

Ankle/foot condition	Prescription orthotics
Patellofemoral pain syndrome	Foot orthoses can be useful if the condition causes excessive pronation of the foot Prefabricated foot orthoses may be prescribed if the patient reports a reduction in pain wearing the orthosis during the single-leg squat or double-leg squat test Duration of use: up to six weeks
Morton's neuroma	Shoe modifications (e.g. wide toe boxes, low heels, metatarsal pads) have around 63% success rate in Morton's neuromas (Saygi *et al.*, 2005) Most commonly prescribed orthotics: metatarsal pads Duration of use: six months
Ankle arthritis	Moulded ankle–foot orthosis has been the mainstay orthosis for ankle arthritis The moulded orthosis can be combined with a rocker-bottom shoe and a cushioned heel to limit and balance motion as much as possible Most commonly prescribed orthotics: Arizona brace, moulded custom orthosis, rocker-bottom shoe, solid ankle cushion heel

Adapted from Elattar et al. (2018)

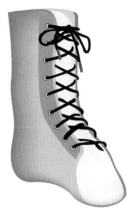

Figure 7.5 Arizona brace

Use of orthotics for overpronation and flatfoot

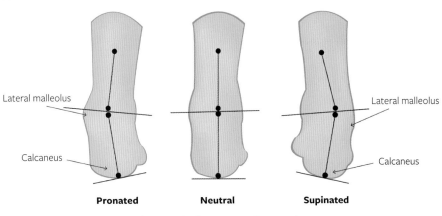

Figure 7.6 Three types of pronation

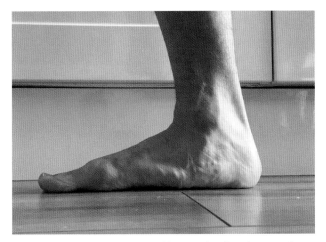

Figure 7.7 Flattening of medial longitudinal arch – pes planus

Pronation is a natural process of the gait cycle that occurs when the arch of the foot rolls inward for weight distribution after landing. However, if there is an excessive inward rolling of the arch, it is called overpronation. This condition is often confused with another condition – flatfoot. Although flatfoot is a different condition with little to no arch while standing, both conditions can occur simultaneously and often expose the lower limb to more ground reaction forces, which ultimately put excessive stress on the affected person's knees and hips. In addition, overpronation can cause early muscle fatigue and eventual straining of the tibia and its periosteum due to the increased anti-pronatory, invertor and plantar flexor muscle activity (Murley *et al.*, 2009; Naderi *et al.*,

2019). In summary, both overpronation and flatfoot may make people more susceptible to specific foot and ankle injuries. These include:

- Achilles tendinopathy

- ankle instability

- heel pain

- posterior tibial tendon dysfunction

- patellofemoral pain syndrome

- hallux valgus

- shin splints

- plantar fasciitis

- stress fractures in the foot.

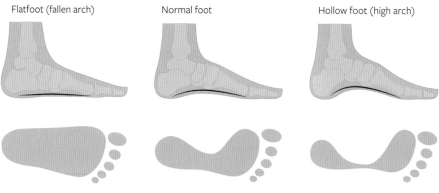

Figure 7.8 Pathologies of the foot

From the above discussion, it can be said that management of overpronation and flatfoot may be an effective means of preventing several foot/ankle injuries. Foot orthoses have long been recommended by physicians and physiotherapists alike to normalise lower-limb kinematics and prevent the foot from overpronating and flattening (Hsu *et al.*, 2014; Naderi *et al.*, 2019). Studies have also reported positive effects of using orthotics for foot or ankle problems such as providing anatomical arch support, normalisation of dynamic foot-pressure distribution, aligning the foot to a neutral position and alteration in muscle activity patterns (Murley *et al.*, 2010; Lo *et al.*, 2016; Bonanno *et al.*, 2017). However, the apparent correction in foot posture with orthotics also has some drawbacks. Because foot orthotics are passive, it is highly likely that the correction in the foot arch does not come from the patient's own muscles. These muscles over time become weak and may potentially impair some of their beneficial functions such as efficient gait and shock absorption (Berengueres *et al.*, 2014; Kelly *et al.*, 2014).

On the other hand, overpronation, flatfoot and similar conditions have been a topic of great controversy among health practitioners of bodywork and movement therapies including physiotherapists, osteopaths, chiropractors and orthotists. Until now, there has been little agreement on the very definition of flatfoot. An agreement still needs to be reached regarding the degree of foot flatness that should be considered a clinically relevant problem and how to measure it simply and correctly (Evans and Rome, 2011; Wallden, 2015). It has also been debated whether overpronation of the foot is associated with increased risk of foot injuries. In fact, only a small effect of association has been found between foot pronation and injury risk (Neal *et al.*, 2014; Nielsen *et al.*, 2014). In reality, the multibillion-dollar sports-shoe industry is mainly responsible for much of the negative marketing against foot pronation and the need to prevent it to avoid injuries (Richards *et al.*, 2009). Pronation is actually a much-needed phase of motion while running. If this phase is prevented, the runner's foot would land with a considerable amount of rigidity and subsequent force, which could eventually lead to disastrous consequences.

In practice, there has been a growing tendency among practitioners to prescribe orthotics and anti-pronation shoes even with the slightest hint of flat feet or overpronation. Such practice needs to be stopped. Practitioners should first carefully assess the degree of overpronation and flatness and then judge whether it might be contributing to a foot injury. They should also examine whether excessive pronation or flatness is the result of muscular weakness or other musculoskeletal problems. In such cases, they should address the problem first before prescribing any orthotics.

References

Aboutorabi, A., Arazpour, M., Bani, M.A., Saeedi, H. and Head, J.S. (2017) Efficacy of ankle foot orthoses types on walking in children with cerebral palsy: A systematic review. *Annals of Physical and Rehabilitation Medicine* 60, 6, 393–402.

Berengueres, J., Fritschi, M. and McClanahan, R. (2014) A smart pressure-sensitive insole that reminds you to walk correctly: An orthotic-less treatment for over pronation. *36th Annual International Conference of the IEEE Engineering in Medicine and Biology Society.* IEEE.

Bonanno, D.R., Landorf, K.B., Munteanu, S.E., Murley, G.S. and Menz, H.B. (2017) Effectiveness of foot orthoses and shock-absorbing insoles for the prevention of injury: A systematic review and meta-analysis. *British Journal of Sports Medicine* 51, 2, 86–96.

Cameron-Fiddes, V. and Santos, D. (2013) The use of 'off-the-shelf' foot orthoses in the reduction of foot symptoms in patients with early rheumatoid arthritis. *The Foot 23*, 4, 123–129.

Choo, Y.J. and Chang, M.C. (2021) Effectiveness of an ankle–foot orthosis on walking in patients with stroke: A systematic review and meta-analysis. *Scientific Reports 11*, 1, 1–12.

Condie, E. (2004) Report of a consensus conference on the orthotic management of stroke patients. *Report of a Consensus Conference on the Orthotic Management of Stroke*. ISPO.

Delafontaine, A., Gagey, O., Colnaghi, S., Do, M.C. and Honeine, J.L. (2017) Rigid ankle foot orthosis deteriorates mediolateral balance control and vertical braking during gait initiation. *Frontiers in Human Neuroscience 11*, 214.

Elattar, O., Smith, T., Ferguson, A., Farber, D. and Wapner, K. (2018) Uses of braces and orthotics for conservative management of foot and ankle disorders. *Foot and Ankle Orthopaedics 3*, 3, https://doi.org/10.1177%2F2473011418780700

Evans, A.M. and Rome, K. (2011) A review of the evidence for non-surgical interventions for flexible pediatric flat feet. *European Journal of Physical and Rehabilitation Medicine 47*, 1, 1–21.

Fisk, J.R., DeMuth, S., Campbell, J., DiBello, T. *et al.* (2016) Suggested guidelines for the prescription of orthotic services, device delivery, education, and follow-up care: A multidisciplinary white paper. *Military Medicine 181*, suppl. 2, 11–17.

Fox, J.R. and Lovegreen, W. (2019) Lower Limb Orthoses. In J. Webster and D. Murphy (eds) *Atlas of Orthoses and Assistive Devices*, 5th edn. Elsevier.

Gross, M.T., Byers, J.M., Krafft, J.L., Lackey, E.J. and Melton, K.M. (2002) The impact of custom semirigid foot orthotics on pain and disability for individuals with plantar fasciitis. *Journal of Orthopaedic and Sports Physical Therapy 32*, 4, 149–157.

Harlaar, J., Brehm, M., Becher, J.G., Bregman, D.J. *et al.* (2010) Studies examining the efficacy of ankle foot orthoses should report activity level and mechanical evidence. *Prosthetics and Orthotics International 34*, 3, 327–335.

Hijmans, J.M. and Geertzen, J.H.B. (2006) Development of clinical guidelines for the prescription of orthoses in patients with neurological disorders in the Netherlands. *Prosthetics and Orthotics International 30*, 1, 35–43.

Hsu, W.H., Lewis, C.L., Monaghan, G.M., Saltzman, E., Hamill, J. and Holt, K.G. (2014) Orthoses posted in both the forefoot and rearfoot reduce moments and angular impulses on lower extremity joints during walking. *Journal of Biomechanics 47*, 11, 2618–2625.

Janisse, D.J. and Janisse, E. (2008) Shoe modification and the use of orthoses in the treatment of foot and ankle pathology. *Journal of the American Academy of Orthopaedic Surgeons 16*, 3, 152–158.

Jarrett, B. and Marcus, R. (2006) *Prescription Custom Foot Orthoses Practice Guidelines*. Bethesda, MD: American College of Foot and Ankle Orthopedics and Medicine.

Jung, D.Y., Koh, E.K. and Kwon, O.Y. (2011) Effect of foot orthoses and short-foot exercise on the cross-sectional area of the abductor hallucis muscle in subjects with pes planus: A randomized controlled trial 1. *Journal of Back and Musculoskeletal Rehabilitation 24*, 4, 225–231.

Kelly, L.A., Cresswell, A.G., Racinais, S., Whiteley, R. and Lichtwark, G. (2014) Intrinsic foot muscles have the capacity to control deformation of the longitudinal arch. *Journal of the Royal Society Interface 11*, 93, 20131188.

Landorf, K.B. and Keenan, A.M. (2000) Efficacy of foot orthoses: What does the literature tell us? *Journal of the American Podiatric Medical Association 90*, 3, 149–158.

Lo, W.T., Wong, D.P., Yick, K.L., Ng, S.P. and Yip, J. (2016) Effects of custom-made textile insoles on plantar pressure distribution and lower limb EMG activity during turning. *Journal of Foot and Ankle Research 9*, 1, 1–13.

Menz, H.B., Allan, J.J., Bonanno, D.R., Landorf, K.B. and Murley, G.S. (2017) Custom-made foot orthoses: An analysis of prescription characteristics from an Australian commercial orthotic laboratory. *Journal of Foot and Ankle Research 10*, 1, 1–9.

Murley, G.S., Landorf, K.B. and Menz, H.B. (2010) Do foot orthoses change lower limb muscle activity in flat-arched feet towards a pattern observed in normal-arched feet? *Clinical Biomechanics 25*, 7, 728–736.

Murley, G.S., Menz, H.B. and Landorf, K.B. (2009) Foot posture influences the electromyographic activity of selected lower limb muscles during gait. *Journal of Foot and Ankle Research 2*, 1, 1–9.

Naderi, A., Degens, H. and Sakinepoor, A. (2019) Arch-support foot-orthoses normalize dynamic in-shoe foot pressure distribution in medial tibial stress syndrome. *European Journal of Sport Science 19*, 2, 247–257.

Neal, B.S., Griffiths, I.B., Dowling, G.J., Murley, G.S. *et al.* (2014) Foot posture as a risk factor for lower limb overuse injury: A systematic review and meta-analysis. *Journal of Foot and Ankle Research 7*, 1, 1–13.

Nielsen, R.O., Buist, I., Parner, E.T., Nohr, E.A. *et al.* (2014) Foot pronation is not associated with increased injury risk in novice runners wearing a neutral shoe: A 1-year prospective cohort study. *British Journal of Sports Medicine 48*, 6, 440–447.

Protopapas, K. and Perry, S.D. (2020) The effect of a 12-week custom foot orthotic intervention on muscle size and muscle activity of the intrinsic foot muscle of young adults during gait termination. *Clinical Biomechanics 78*, 105063.

Richards, C.E., Magin, P.J. and Callister, R. (2009) Is your prescription of distance running shoes evidence-based? *British Journal of Sports Medicine 43*, 3, 159–162.

Ridgewell, E., Dobson, F., Bach, T. and Baker, R. (2010) A systematic review to determine best practice reporting guidelines for AFO interventions in studies involving children with cerebral palsy. *Prosthetics and Orthotics International 34*, 2, 129–145.

Saygi, B., Yildirim, Y., Saygi, E.K., Kara, H. and Esemenli, T. (2005) Morton neuroma: Comparative results of two conservative methods. *Foot and Ankle International 26*, 7, 556–559.

Tran, K. and Spry, C. (2019) *Custom-Made Foot Orthoses versus Prefabricated Foot Orthoses: A Review of Clinical Effectiveness and Cost-Effectiveness* [Internet]. Ottawa: Canadian Agency for Drugs and Technologies in Health, www.ncbi.nlm.nih.gov/books/NBK549527

Wallden, M. (2015) Don't get caught flat footed: How over-pronation may just be a dysfunctional model. *Journal of Bodywork and Movement Therapies 19*, 2, 357–361.

Willy, R.W., Hoglund, L.T., Barton, C.J., Bolgla, L.A. *et al.* (2019) Patellofemoral pain: Clinical practice guidelines linked to the International Classification of Functioning, Disability and Health from the Academy of Orthopaedic Physical Therapy of the American Physical Therapy Association. *Journal of Orthopaedic and Sports Physical Therapy 49*, 9, CPG1–CPG95.

Chapter 8

Bunions – Manual Therapy and Surgical Referral

DR KUMAR KUNASINGAM

This chapter is of personal interest to me as a specialist in foot and ankle surgery and in minimal invasive surgical procedures for the treatment of hallux valgus issues, through the publication of research on the very best standards of care and from years of specialist training.

Although we won't be going into the intricacies of this common condition in depth, I hope to give you an overview of the condition, myths around development, treatment and how we can work together as physical therapists and surgical consultants. The cliché 'Teamwork makes the dream work' is actually not far from the truth, and through interprofessional cooperation and education we can deliver the very best of patient care. So let's start on the deep dive into bunions!

A bunion, also called hallux valgus (HV), is a common deformity of the forefoot. It is characterised by a medial eminence in the form of a prominent bump on the inside of the foot. The deformity usually forms when the first metatarsophalangeal (MTP) joint moves out of its normal alignment, causing the first metatarsal bone to deviate medially and the hallux to deviate laterally towards the second toe. A bunion often develops slowly, with progressive increase in the size of the deformity. It gradually changes the normal structure of metatarsal bone, forming a bony bump. The HV deformity can, at times, become red, swollen and painful, causing difficulty performing daily activities. These symptoms often worsen if the patient wears ill-fitting shoes, especially those with a narrow toe box (Wülker and Mittag, 2012; Hecht and Lin, 2014).

Epidemiologically, HV is a highly prevalent forefoot deformity, particularly in adult females. This may be due to the more flexible soft tissues they have and/or the differences in osseous anatomy compared with men (Ferrari *et al.*, 2004; Nguyen *et al.*, 2010; Choi *et al.*, 2015). The deformity affects about 35% of adults over 65 years of age, up to 23% of those between 18 and 65 years old and around 8% of children below 18 years (Nix *et al.*, 2010). In the United Kingdom, HV is estimated to affect about 28.4% of adults over 30 years of age (Roddy *et al.*, 2008). The exact aetiology of this deformity remains undetermined. Multiple contributing factors are thought to play a role in its origin, including type of footwear, genetic predisposition, arthritis, gastrocnemius equinus, foot skeletal variations (e.g. pes planovalgus, forefoot varus, short first metatarsal) and abnormal foot mechanics (Coughlin and Jones, 2007). However, evidence to support these associations is still limited. As a result, there exist many misconceptions about the aetiology and treatment of HV.

In most cases, conservative treatments (e.g. manual therapy, shoe modifications, orthotics, night splints) are first trialled to reduce HV symptoms. Surgery is often reserved for those who continue to have painful symptoms despite appropriate non-surgical management. With surgical management, the bony union usually occurs within 6–7 weeks after the surgery (Blitz *et al.*, 2010). There are, however, over 100 different open bony and soft-tissue surgical procedures to correct HV. Each of these techniques has its own advantages and disadvantages. The decision to select a suitable technique therefore primarily depends on the severity and extent of the deformity and the variations in forefoot skeletal alignment (Fraissler *et al.*, 2016). More recently, minimally invasive procedures such as chevron Akin have been introduced, which demonstrate effective pain relief in clinical studies (Holme *et al.*, 2020). These techniques are gaining popularity due to the potential for reduced surgical time, smaller scar size and greater early postoperative movement compared with open osteotomy. However, there are two major drawbacks of these techniques: high complication rates and lack of adequate evidence (Redfern and Perera, 2014).

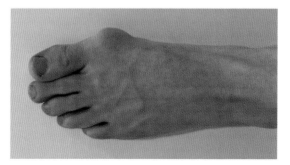

Figure 8.1 Bunion 1

This chapter is written to dispel some of the common misconceptions about HV and discuss its treatment strategies including non-invasive management, surgical referral, minimally invasive surgery and postoperative rehabilitation.

Common misconceptions about bunions

Misconception 1: High heels are a primary causative factor for HV in women

There is evidence that ill-fitting shoes can exacerbate HV symptoms in women and may play a role in the progression of certain foot pathologies (Ikpeze *et al.*, 2015). This is because the narrow toe box and high heel of these shoes displace the centre of gravity of the foot. Hence, in patients with HV, wearing these shoes can be an aggravating factor for the increase in pain and other symptoms. However, this does not make wearing high heels or tight shoes a primary cause of HV. In fact, no study has so far presented solid evidence to prove an association between the development of a bunion and wearing a high-heel shoe (Yu *et al.*, 2020). There are many women who regularly wear tight, high-heel shoes but have no HV deformity (Kuhn and Alvi, 2020). Nevertheless, it is always better to wear appropriate footwear, particularly shoes with wider toe boxes and flatter heels.

Misconception 2: Non–invasive treatment can truly fix a bunion

There is currently little to no research-based evidence to support a clinically significant correction of HV with non-surgical interventions. In fact, most experts agree that non-surgical management of HV cannot correct the deformity but is highly effective to relieve the symptoms (Fraissler *et al.*, 2016; Hurn *et al.*, 2016; Kuhn and Alvi, 2020). In addition, a meta-analysis published by Hurn *et al.* (2021) also concluded that only a low level of evidence currently exists to support the effectiveness of non-surgical management of HV. The authors, however, reported a significant reduction in pain with multiple non-surgical options including foot orthoses, dynamic and night splints, manual therapy, Botox injections and multifaceted physical therapies.

Misconception 3: Bunions are similar to gout

Bunions are often confused with gout due to the similarity in symptoms, the affected joint (i.e. the first MTP joint) and appearance. Both conditions primarily affect the hallux and can cause the MTP joint to become red and swollen (Becker and Childress, 2018). However, aside from these similarities, they are totally two different conditions with distinct aetiology and pathophysiology. Gout is a complex type of arthritis that usually results from the build-up of uric acid in the blood. The increase in uric acid eventually leads to the production of urate crystals, which cause intense pain in the joint (Schumacher, 2008). In contrast, as discussed above, a bunion or HV is more of a mechanical issue that often results from direct pressure into the MTP joint. Nevertheless, some recent studies have also reported a high prevalence of HV in patients with gout, particularly in those requiring urate-lowering therapy (Roddy *et al.*, 2014; Blandin *et al.*, 2016; Blandin *et al.*, 2018).

Misconception 4: HV cannot be fully reversed

Recurrence of the bony bump is indeed a common complication after corrective surgery. In general, rates of HV recurrence have been reported to vary between 2.7% and 16% in the literature (Lehman, 2003; Robinson and Limbers, 2005; Kilmartin and O'Kane, 2010; Okuda *et al.*, 2011). However, these rates differ based on the reconstructive procedure performed. In addition, both surgical and patient-related factors (e.g. technical competency of the surgeon, appropriateness of the applied procedure, medical comorbidities of the patient) play a role in the recurrence of HV. Taken together, a well-chosen and appropriately performed procedure can lead to a long-term correction without recurrence (Raikin *et al.*, 2014).

Non-invasive management

Non-invasive management of HV is primarily aimed at managing symptoms. Although proponents of various non-surgical options claim them to be effective, there is currently no research-based evidence that recommends their use for the correction of the actual bunion deformity (Kuhn and Alvi, 2020). However, the consensus statement by the American College of Foot and Ankle Surgeons still supports the use of non-invasive treatments prior to operative management (Vanore *et al.*, 2003). In fact, in most cases with mild to moderate HV, periodic evaluation of the deformity is all that's needed. The deformity should be checked both clinically and radiologically to determine the progression of the HV and the need for non-surgical management (Fraissler *et al.*, 2016). Non-invasive treatment options that may be trialled include the following:

- **Shoe modification:** It is important for patients with HV to wear the right type of shoes. Most experts often recommend low-heeled shoes with a wide toe box that fit properly and do not put any pressure on the bunion. Sometimes, patients may need further modification to their shoes. For example, a stretcher may be used to stretch out the toe areas so that there is enough space. However, if the patient develops other severe deformity such as hammer toes or claw toes, surgical referral should be made (Wülker and Mittag, 2012).

- **Orthotic devices:** Use of orthotics in patients with HV can help relieve pressure off the bunion, improve alignment of the hallux and provide alleviation of symptoms. A wide range of orthotic devices are used for HV management including shoe insoles, night splints, toe spacers and toe straighteners, to name a few (Becker and Childress, 2018).

  ○ Insoles have long been suggested to be useful for metatarsalgia management (Stinus and Weber, 2005).

  ○ Wearing a night splint can help move the hallux medially; however, this is only possible while the skeleton is still growing. Once skeletal growth ends, it can only alleviate symptoms (Wülker and Mittag, 2012).

  ○ Toe spacers or straighteners can help reduce pressure on the hallux by keeping it in a correct position (Tehraninasr *et al.*, 2008).

- **Padding:** Bunion pads over the medial eminence can help prevent irritation by cushioning the painful area. These are readily available in pharmacies. However, the patient should first trial the pad for a short period. If it is not that helpful, they should avoid it as its size may increase the pressure on the bunion and eventually worsen the pain (Park and Chang, 2019).

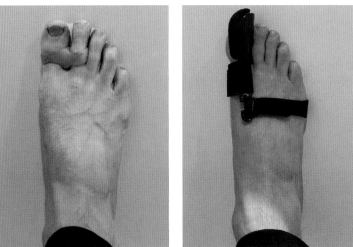

Figure 8.2 Toe corrector   *Figure 8.3 Toe separator*

- **Manual therapy:** Manual therapists can help assist patients with HV to maintain mobility and strength in the affected MTP joint both before and after surgery. They help patients in the selection of the right type of orthotic devices, assessing gait on the affected side. Preoperatively, the goal of this therapy is to ensure safe, controlled movements with assistive devices, muscle strengthening and functional training. Post-operatively, manual therapists assist patients to regain motion and strength in the affected joint during the course of the rehabilitation process (Mortka and Lisiński, 2015).

- **Pharmacotherapy:** Common analgesics such as acetaminophen and nonsteroidal anti-inflammatory drugs (NSAIDs) (e.g. naproxen and ketorolac) are frequently prescribed for HV management to relieve pain and reduce swelling and inflammation. The use of corticosteroid injections in HV treatment is rare. They are typically indicated if there is an inflamed bursa with the bunion. Recently, Wu *et al.* (2015) evaluated the effects of botulinum toxin (type A) injection on painful HV and reported that the toxin significantly improved pain scores, disability scores and HV angle compared with the control. However, more research is needed to establish it as a conservative treatment.

Special considerations for non-surgical care

Surgical intervention for HV is not recommended for all patient groups. It should be avoided in the presence of an absolute contraindication such as arterial occlusive disease, as it can result in decreased perfusion (Williams *et al.*, 2006). In addition, juvenile HV should be treated with non-surgical management. This is because as the skeleton is still growing in this patient population, there is a high possibility of recurrence after the surgery. On the other hand, it is possible to correct juvenile HV with assistive devices (Chell and Dhar, 2014).

A non-invasive approach should also be considered if the patient presents with any of the following conditions:

- neuromuscular disorders
- ligamentous laxity
- general hypermobility
- chronic polyarthritis
- rheumatic diseases
- diabetes.

Surgical referral

In determining the need for surgical management, radiographic imaging is not essential and often plays a less significant role. Surgical referral for HV is usually made in the following clinical scenarios:

- the pain persists even after weeks of various non-surgical treatments
- the pain regularly interferes with the activities of daily living
- the pain markedly impairs the affected limb function.

Note: It is not a requisite that the hallux will always be involved with the bunion pain. The pain can initially arise from other digits, which may manifest as hammer or claw toes. However, even in such a case, surgical correction should be indicated for both the smaller toes and the HV (Wülker and Mittag, 2012).

In the surgical management of HV, however, radiographic measurements can help to determine the degree of bunion deformity. In general, a patient is considered to have a HV deformity if there exists an angle of more than

15° between the axis of the first metatarsal shaft and the proximal phalanx of the first toe (Hecht and Lin, 2014). Table 8.1 presents radiologically relevant angular measurements of the HV deformity.

Table 8.1 Radiographic measurements of the HV deformity

Radiological measures	Degree
HV angle (angle between the first metatarsal bone and the proximal phalanx of the hallux)	15–20° (mild)
	21–39° (moderate)
	≥ 40° (severe)
Intermetatarsal angle (angle between the first two metatarsals)	> 9° (pathological)
HV interphalangeus angle (the metaphyseal-diaphyseal angle of the first proximal phalanx)	> 10° (pathological)

Sources: Coughlin and Freund (2001); Hecht and Lin (2014)

Operative techniques

The success of an HV surgery depends largely on the specific operative technique used to treat the individual deformity. Various factors play a role in the selection of a surgical procedure, including the presence of arthritis, the characteristics of the patient (e.g. age, sex, activity level), the severity and extent of the deformity, variations in forefoot skeletal alignment, experience and command of the surgeon in operative techniques, and the preference of the surgeon (Fraissler *et al.*, 2016; Kuhn and Alvi, 2020). As discussed above, there are more than 100 different HV correction procedures described in the literature. However, almost all of these operative techniques involve one of the following basic approaches:

- **Osteotomy:** The term 'osteotomy' simply means 'bone cutting'. In this surgical procedure, the surgeon makes a cut in the first metatarsal bone under general anaesthesia to realign it into a less adducted position. The size and location of bone cutting primarily depend on the specific osteotomy procedure selected by the surgeon. There are many different types of HV osteotomies. Some of the most commonly used techniques include Wilson osteotomy, chevron osteotomy, scarf osteotomy, Ludloff osteotomy, Moberg osteotomy, Akin osteotomy and Mann osteotomy (Trnka, 2005; Kuhn and Alvi, 2020).

- **Arthroplasty:** Also known as joint replacement surgery, this surgical procedure is usually performed to restore the function of the MTP joint. Arthroplasty of HV involves removal of part of the damaged or arthritic MTP joint and replacing it with an implant or prosthesis. There are both full and partial joint arthroplasty for the correction of HV deformity. Partial replacement or hemiarthroplasty requires less bone resection and does not reduce the toe length. The most common example of resection arthroplasty is the Keller resection arthroplasty, which is primarily indicated only in elderly and inactive patients. This is due to its high complication rate in younger patients (Machacek *et al.*, 2004; Alarcón *et al.*, 2017).

- **Arthrodesis:** This surgical procedure corrects the position of the MTP joint through fusion of the hallux with the metatarsal bone. The procedure is usually reserved for elderly patients with severe HV or MTP joint osteoarthritis. Unlike resection arthroplasty, MTP arthrodesis can be indicated to patients with very pronounced HV deformities and a high level of physical activity. The most likely reason for this is that arthrodesis allows for a firm contact of the hallux with the surface during heel rise. Other advantages of this technique include improved ambulation, preserved function, high bone fusion rate and fewer complications. Downsides of arthrodesis are joint stiffness, metatarsalgia and fewer footwear alternatives (Wülker and Mittag, 2012; Perugia *et al.*, 2017; Kuhn and Alvi, 2020).

- **Soft-tissue procedures:** There are various soft-tissue procedures to correct HV; however, most are now abandoned due to potential complications. The one procedure that is currently in use is the modified McBride procedure, also called the distal soft-tissue procedure. It has proven to be an effective adjunct to distal metatarsal osteotomies for HV correction. The modified McBride procedure aims to realign the proximal phalanx with the metatarsal head by releasing the adductor hallucis, the sesamoid ligaments and the lateral joint capsule (Lui *et al.*, 2005; Schneider, 2013).

Minimally invasive surgical procedures

Over the last decade, there has been an increase in the popularity of minimally invasive techniques for HV correction. As discussed above, this has been primarily due to the theoretical potential for reduced surgical time, smaller scar size, less soft-tissue trauma and faster recovery. Currently, several minimally invasive techniques are used for HV correction, including percutaneous osteotomy, minimum incision osteotomy and arthroscopy. The earliest of these techniques is the percutaneous surgery, which was pioneered in the form of subcapital osteotomy, Reverdin–Isham procedure and variants thereof during the 1990s. The early success and growing popularity of these techniques actually paved the way for second-generation minimally invasive techniques during the 2000s (Isham, 1991; Bösch *et al.*, 2000; Maffulli *et al.*, 2011).

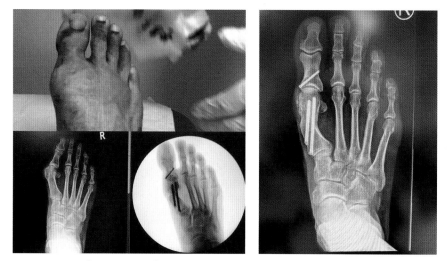

Figure 8.4 Bunion 2   *Figure 8.5 Bunion 3*

First and second generations of the minimally invasive HV procedures involved metatarsal osteotomies without any fixation or with Kirschner wire fixation or rigid internal (screw) fixation. For mild to moderate HV deformity, the average correction of HV angle with these techniques has been reported to improve about 16.4° postoperatively, and for moderate to severe HV around 28.3°. The correction in intermetatarsal angle with these techniques is reported to improve up to 6° postoperatively (Bia *et al.*, 2018). However, these techniques have been highly criticised in the literature for high complication rates and lack of adequate evidence. In fact, there is currently too little evidence to recommend manually invasive techniques over traditional procedures for HV correction. In addition, the complication rate has been reported to range from 13% to 19% (Bia *et al.*, 2018; Malagelada *et al.*, 2019).

The most recent of these minimally invasive techniques is the third-generation chevron Akin osteotomy (Redfern and Perera, 2014). According to a recent systematic review by Malagelada *et al.* (2019), this technique has been shown to have the most potential for correcting the HV angle. Although good evidence has been presented from originator centres supporting this technique (Perera *et al.*, 2015; Redfern *et al.*, 2015), there has been little evidence up to now from non-originator surgeons. Recently, a non-originator group led by Holme *et al.* (2020) conducted a case series on 40 consecutive HV patients undergoing chevron Akin osteotomy. The authors used a validated measure to evaluate patient-reported outcome and followed up all included patients for an average of 12 months. They reported a complication rate of only 10% following the surgery but a 100% positive patient-reported outcome at 12 months. No recurrences or other complications were reported at 12 months. Nevertheless, further research, particularly long-term randomised controlled trials, is needed to assess the true efficacy of minimally invasive HV procedures.

Rehabilitation

Postoperative care or rehabilitation varies from person to person depending on the type of invasive procedure performed and the nature and extent of the HV deformity (Wülker and Mittag, 2012; Fraissler *et al.*, 2016). In general, however, the following protocol is adhered to in most cases:

- full weight-bearing mobilisation in a flat shoe with stiff sole for six weeks

- full weight-bearing with mobility aids (e.g. walker or crutches) for balance and support, if needed

- general instructions to avoid swelling, such as keeping the operated foot raised during the first two weeks

- referral to a physiotherapist or a manual therapist before discharge

- mild stretching exercises and hands-on techniques by the therapist to improve ankle range of motion after two weeks

- stretching, strengthening exercises, joint mobilisation and gait training by the therapist from six weeks onwards.

References

Alarcón, L.L.D., Arroyo, G.D. and Muñoz, P.A.D. (2017) Keller arthroplasty vs hemi-implant arthroplasty for the surgical treatment of hallux rigidus: Mid-term comparative analysis. *Revista Española de Podología* 28, 1, e9–e17.

Becker, B.A. and Childress, M.A. (2018) Common foot problems: Over-the-counter treatments and home care. *American Family Physician* 98, 5, 298–303.

Bia, A., Guerra-Pinto, F., Pereira, B.S., Corte-Real, N. and Oliva, X.M. (2018) Percutaneous osteotomies in hallux valgus: A systematic review. *The Journal of Foot and Ankle Surgery* 57, 1, 123–130.

Blandin, C., Forien, M., Dieudé, P. and Ottaviani, S. (2016) AB0827 high prevalence of hallux valgus in gouty patients requiring urate lowering therapy. *Annals of the Rheumatic Diseases* 75, 2, 1186.

Blandin, C., Forien, M., Gardette, A., Palazzo, E., Dieudé, P. and Ottaviani, S. (2018) Tophus size is associated with hallux valgus deformity in gout. *European Journal of Clinical Investigation* 48, 1, e12862.

Blitz, N.M., Lee, T., Williams, K., Barkan, H. and DiDimenico, L.A. (2010) Early weight bearing after modified lapidus arthodesis: A multicenter review of 80 cases. *The Journal of Foot and Ankle Surgery* 49, 4, 357–362.

Bösch, P., Wanke, S. and Legenstein, R. (2000) Hallux valgus correction by the method of Bösch: A new technique with a seven-to-ten-year follow-up. *Foot and Ankle Clinics* 5, 3, 485–498.

Chell, J. and Dhar, S. (2014) Pediatric hallux valgus. *Foot and Ankle Clinics* 19, 2, 235–243.

Choi, G.W., Kim, H.J., Kim, T.W., Lee, J.W., Park, S.B. and Kim, J.K. (2015) Sex-related differences in outcomes after hallux valgus surgery. *Yonsei Medical Journal* 56, 2, 466–473.

Coughlin, M.J. and Freund, E. (2001) The reliability of angular measurements in hallux valgus deformities. *Foot and Ankle International* 22, 5, 369–379.

Coughlin, M.J. and Jones, C.P. (2007) Hallux valgus: Demographics, etiology, and radiographic assessment. *Foot and Ankle International* 28, 7, 759–777.

Ferrari, J., Hopkinson, D.A. and Linney, A.D. (2004) Size and shape differences between male and female foot bones: Is the female foot predisposed to hallux abducto valgus deformity? *Journal of the American Podiatric Medical Association* 94, 5, 434–452.

Fraissler, L., Konrads, C., Hoberg, M., Rudert, M. and Walcher, M. (2016) Treatment of hallux valgus deformity. *EFORT Open Reviews* 1, 8, 295–302.

Hecht, P.J. and Lin, T.J. (2014) Hallux valgus. *Medical Clinics* 98, 2, 227–232.

Holme, T.J., Sivaloganathan, S.S., Patel, B. and Kunasingam, K. (2020) Third-generation minimally invasive chevron Akin osteotomy for hallux valgus. *Foot and Ankle International* 41, 1, 50–56.

Hurn, S.E., Matthews, B.G., Munteanu, S.E. and Menz, H.B. (2021) Effectiveness of non-surgical interventions for hallux valgus: A systematic review and meta-analysis. *Arthritis Care and Research*, https://doi.org/10.1002/acr.24603

Hurn, S.E., Vicenzino, B.T. and Smith, M.D. (2016) Non-surgical treatment of hallux valgus: A current practice survey of Australian podiatrists. *Journal of Foot and Ankle Research* 9, 1, 1–9.

Ikpeze, T.C., Omar, A. and Elfar, J.H. (2015) Evaluating problems with footwear in the geriatric population. *Geriatric Orthopaedic Surgery and Rehabilitation* 6, 4, 338–340.

Isham, S.A. (1991) The Reverdin-Isham procedure for the correction of hallux abducto valgus: A distal metatarsal osteotomy procedure. *Clinics in Podiatric Medicine and Surgery* 8, 1, 81–94.

Kilmartin, T.E. and O'Kane, C. (2010) Combined rotation scarf and Akin osteotomies for hallux valgus: A patient focussed 9 year follow up of 50 patients. *Journal of Foot and Ankle Research* 3, 1, 1–12.

Kuhn, J. and Alvi, F. (2020) Hallux Valgus. StatPearls [Internet], www.ncbi.nlm.nih.gov/books/NBK553092

Lehman, D.E. (2003) Salvage of complications of hallux valgus surgery. *Foot and Ankle Clinics* 8, 1, 15–35.

Lui, T.H., Ng, S. and Chan, K.B. (2005) Endoscopic distal soft tissue procedure in hallux valgus surgery. *Arthroscopy: The Journal of Arthroscopic and Related Surgery* 21, 11, 1403.

Machacek Jr, F., Easley, M.E., Gruber, F., Ritschl, P. and Trnka, H.J. (2004) Salvage of a failed Keller resection arthroplasty. *Journal of Bone and Joint Surgery* 86, 6, 1131–1138.

Maffulli, N., Longo, U.G., Marinozzi, A. and Denaro, V. (2011) Hallux valgus: Effectiveness and safety of minimally invasive surgery. A systematic review. *British Medical Bulletin* 97, 1, 149–167.

Malagelada, F., Sahirad, C., Dalmau-Pastor, M., Vega, J. *et al.* (2019) Minimally invasive surgery for hallux valgus: A systematic review of current surgical techniques. *International Orthopaedics* 43, 3, 625–637.

Mortka, K. and Lisiński, P. (2015) Hallux valgus – a case for a physiotherapist or only for a surgeon? Literature review. *Journal of Physical Therapy Science* 27, 10, 3303–3307.

Nguyen, U.S., Hillstrom, H.J., Li, W., Dufour, A.B. *et al.* (2010) Factors associated with hallux valgus in a population-based study of older women and men: The MOBILIZE Boston Study. *Osteoarthritis and Cartilage* 18, 1, 41–46.

Nix, S., Smith, M. and Vicenzino, B. (2010) Prevalence of hallux valgus in the general population: A systematic review and meta-analysis. *Journal of Foot and Ankle Research* 3, 1, 1–9.

Okuda, R., Kinoshita, M., Yasuda, T., Jotoku, T., Shima, H. and Takamura, M. (2011) Hallux valgus angle as a predictor of recurrence following proximal metatarsal osteotomy. *Journal of Orthopaedic Science* 16, 6, 760–764.

Park, C.H. and Chang, M.C. (2019) Forefoot disorders and conservative treatment. *Yeungnam University Journal of Medicine* 36, 2, 92–98.

Perera, A., Singh, D. and Lomax, A. (2015) Minimally invasive forefoot surgery. *Journal of Trauma and Orthopaedics* 3, 1, 50–54.

Perugia, D., Calderaro, C., Iorio, C., Civintenga, C. *et al.* (2017) Metatarsophalangeal joint arthrodesis for severe hallux valgus in elderly patients. *Journal of the American Academy of Orthopaedic Surgeons* 25, 8, 600.

Raikin, S.M., Miller, A.G. and Daniel, J. (2014) Recurrence of hallux valgus: A review. *Foot and Ankle Clinics* 19, 2, 259–274.

Redfern, D. and Perera, A.M. (2014) Minimally invasive osteotomies. *Foot and Ankle Clinics* 19, 2, 181–189.

Redfern, D., Vernois, J. and Legré, B.P. (2015) Percutaneous surgery of the forefoot. *Clinics in Podiatric Medicine and Surgery* 32, 3, 291–332.

Robinson, A.H.N. and Limbers, J.P. (2005) Modern concepts in the treatment of hallux valgus. *The Journal of Bone and Joint Surgery* 87, 8, 1038–1045.

Roddy, E., Muller, S., Rome, K., Chandratre, P. *et al.* (2014) Chronic foot problems in people with gout: An observational study in primary care. *Rheumatology* 53, 163–163.

Roddy, E., Zhang, W. and Doherty, M. (2008) Prevalence and associations of hallux valgus in a primary care population. *Arthritis Care and Research: Official Journal of the American College of Rheumatology* 59, 6, 857–862.

Schneider, W. (2013) Distal soft tissue procedure in hallux valgus surgery: Biomechanical background and technique. *International Orthopaedics* 37, 9, 1669–1675.

Schumacher Jr, H.R. (2008) The pathogenesis of gout. *Cleveland Clinic Journal of Medicine* 75, S2–4.

Stinus, H. and Weber, F. (2005) Inserts for foot deformities. *Der Orthopade* 34, 8, 776–778.

Tehraninasr, A., Saeedi, H., Forogh, B., Bahramizadeh, M. and Keyhani, M.R. (2008) Effects of insole with toe-separator and night splint on patients with painful hallux valgus: A comparative study. *Prosthetics and Orthotics International* 32, 1, 79–83.

Trnka, H.J. (2005) Osteotomies for hallux valgus correction. *Foot and Ankle Clinics* 10, 1, 15–33.

Vanore, J.V., Christensen, J.C., Kravitz, S.R., Schuberth, J.M. *et al.* (2003) Diagnosis and treatment of first metatarsophalangeal joint disorders. Section 1: Hallux valgus. *The Journal of Foot and Ankle Surgery 42,* 3, 112–123.

Williams, D.T., Price, P. and Harding, K.G. (2006) The influence of diabetes and lower limb arterial disease on cutaneous foot perfusion. *Journal of Vascular Surgery 44,* 4, 770–775.

Wu, K.P.H., Chen, C.K., Lin, S.C., Pei, Y.C. *et al.* (2015) Botulinum Toxin type A injections for patients with painful hallux valgus: A double-blind, randomized controlled study. *Clinical Neurology and Neurosurgery 129,* S58–S62.

Wülker, N. and Mittag, F. (2012) The treatment of hallux valgus. *Deutsches Ärzteblatt International 109,* 49, 857.

Yu, G., Fan, Y., Fan, Y., Li, R. *et al.* (2020) The role of footwear in the pathogenesis of hallux valgus: A proof-of-concept finite element analysis in recent humans and homo naledi. *Frontiers in Bioengineering and Biotechnology 8,* 648.

Chapter 9

Management of Acute Injuries with PEACE and LOVE

IAIN BARROWMAN

Management of acute injuries is complex. Up to now, various acronyms or protocols have been utilised to guide the management, including ICE, RICE, POLICE and PRICE, to name a few. However, there is much more complexity in the clinical management of soft-tissue injuries (Bleakley *et al.*, 2012; Wang and Ni, 2021). Clinicians more often than not have conflicting views about the clinical best practice for the desired treatment outcomes. The primary reason for this is the fact that most of the well-known approaches focus solely on acute management. In addition, while some of the protocols focus on rest and protection to avoid further damage, others give more emphasis on rehabilitation programmes to facilitate faster tissue healing and early recovery. However, none of these protocols outlines a proper guideline for the management and rehabilitation of subacute and chronic stages of tissue healing (Dubois and Esculier, 2020; Wang and Ni, 2021).

In a recent editorial, Dubois and Esculier (2020) came up with two new acronyms, PEACE and LOVE, to encompass the entire rehabilitation continuum. The acronym PEACE addresses the immediate care part of the soft-tissue recovery, while LOVE outlines subsequent management of subacute and chronic injuries. These two acronyms also highlight the need for patient education, the harms of using anti-inflammatories and the importance of taking psychosocial factors into consideration. These add-ons are usually not included in the standard protocols of soft-tissue injuries but can be helpful to enhance recovery.

This chapter aims to discuss what PEACE and LOVE stand for and how they can optimise soft-tissue recovery.

PEACE

The acronym PEACE aims to guide the recovery of soft tissue immediately after an injury, without allowing any further harm. The protocol follows a similar process to the PRICE protocol but with emphasis on making the patient more independent through education on the injury. The PEACE approach is generally carried out for 1–3 days following the injury. However, this timeframe largely depends on the patient's SIN factor, pain levels and mobility. As always, a thorough subjective and objective assessment must be performed to screen for possible red flags or any considerations.

P stands for Protection

- Unload the affected area or limit any aggravating movements for 1–3 days.

- Keep rest to a minimum.

- Let pain signals guide the duration of protection and reloading.

Clinical reasoning: Unloading and restricting activities is suggested to reduce bleeding and swelling, protect the injured fibres from distension and minimise the risk of any further damage to the tissue. Prolonged rest should be avoided as this can affect tissue strength and quality (Bleakley *et al.*, 2012).

E stands for Elevation

- Elevate the affected limb above the level of the heart.

Clinical reasoning: The limb should be elevated to avoid the build-up of interstitial fluid around the affected area and promote the flow of fluid out of tissues. Although there is a lack of evidence in support of elevation, it encompasses a low risk-benefit ratio (Doherty *et al.*, 2017).

A stands for Avoid Anti-Inflammatories

- Avoid anti-inflammatory medications.

- Avoid the use of ice or cryotherapy.

Clinical reasoning: Our bodies naturally undergo various inflammatory processes for the optimal repair and regeneration of injured soft tissues. These phases of healing need to cycle through without interruption and be allowed to play out in full. Should this not happen, the entire healing process may be affected. The use of anti-inflammatory medications impairs the natural tissue-healing mechanism by inhibiting inflammation (Vuurberg *et al.*, 2018). This may also negatively impact the tissue-healing process in the long run, particularly when larger doses are utilised (Ziltener *et al.*, 2010; Lisowska *et al.*, 2018). Hence, the use of this group of medications should be avoided.

The use of ice therapy is another controversial subject in the injury rehabilitation continuum. Although it is known to induce analgesia, no high-quality evidence currently supports its usage in the management of soft-tissue injuries. In addition, cryotherapy can potentially impair the inflammatory process, decrease tissue metabolism, reduce hematoma formation, disrupt revascularisation, delay neutrophil and macrophage infiltration and promote immature myofibres (Singh *et al.*, 2017; Wang and Ni, 2021).

C stands for Compression

- Use taping or bandages to provide an external mechanical compression.

Clinical reasoning: The use of taping or bandages helps restrict intra-articular swelling and tissue haemorrhage. Although the current evidence is conflicting in support of compression, taping or strapping appears to be beneficial in patients with an ankle sprain (Hansrani *et al.*, 2015; Trofa *et al.*, 2020; Nunes *et al.*, 2021).

E stands for Education

- Educate injured patients about the many benefits of adopting an active approach for their recovery.

- Provide better education to patients on their condition and load management.

- Assist patients to set realistic expectations about the time it will take them to recover.

Clinical reasoning: There are many benefits of adopting an active approach over a passive modality. Active protocols often have more significant effects on pain and function immediately after the injury than a passive one. Early passive approaches may also have a negative effect on the injury in the long run (Doherty *et al.*, 2017; Vuurberg *et al.*, 2018). In fact, if therapists nurture patients' locus of control, this can ultimately lead to therapy-dependent behaviour. Hence, better patient education is necessary to avoid the need for unnecessary modalities (e.g. injections or surgery) or overtreatment of the injury. Therapists should also help patients to set realistic expectations about their recovery times, so that they do not go all-out for a 'magic cure'-type approach (Chinn and Hertel, 2010; Lewis and O'Sullivan, 2018).

LOVE

Once the injured soft tissues are addressed with the PEACE approach for the first few days, the LOVE acronym then optimises the subsequent management and rehabilitation.

L stands for Load

- Follow an active approach that incorporates movement and exercise.

- Add early mechanical stress to the injured area if symptoms allow.

- Resume normal activities of daily living as soon as symptoms allow.

Clinical reasoning: An active approach is often beneficial for patients with foot and ankle injuries. At the early stage, optimal loading (without exacerbating symptoms) can help to promote the repair and remodelling of soft tissues and often leads to a process called mechanotransduction, which improves the tolerance of tissues and the capacity of muscles, tendons and ligaments (Khan and Scott, 2009).

O stands for Optimism

- Stay realistic but instil optimistic beliefs and expectations in the heart of the injured patients.

Clinical reasoning: Our brain plays a more important role in how we experience symptoms after an injury than the actual level of damage. Several psychological factors (e.g. fear, depression, catastrophising) can become barriers to recovery. Research has shown that patients displaying such behaviours harm their overall rehabilitation process (Lin *et al.*, 2020). In contrast, optimism is a key factor in a successful rehabilitation programme. Therefore, realistic but optimistic expectations are essential for better treatment outcomes and prognosis. This is because they help instil positive beliefs and thoughts in the patient, and also promote positive behavioural changes (Bialosky *et al.*, 2010; Briet *et al.*, 2016).

V stands for Vascularisation

- Start pain-free cardiovascular exercise such as aerobics a few days after the injury.

Clinical reasoning: Cardiovascular activity is a vital component in the management of lower-limb injuries. It helps to improve oxygen and nutrient supply to the injured area and boost the morale of the affected patient (Lin *et al.*, 2020). The introduction of therapeutic exercise and early mobilisation can benefit patients with foot or ankle injuries by improving physical function, reducing the need for analgesics and facilitating return to work (Chinn and Hertel, 2010; Wagemans *et al.*, 2022).

E stands for Exercise

- Approach exercising using pain as a guide.

- Start with low-impact exercise and gradually increase the level of effort.

Clinical reasoning: A high level of evidence currently supports the use of exercise for the management of foot or ankle injuries. Exercises have been shown to restore strength, mobility and proprioception in the early days following an injury. They also help to prevent the risk of recurrent injuries

(Vuurberg *et al.*, 2018; Wagemans *et al.*, 2022). However, to ensure optimal repairing of the injured structures, patients should avoid pain-aggravating exercises/movements during the subacute phase of recovery (Dubois and Esculier, 2020).

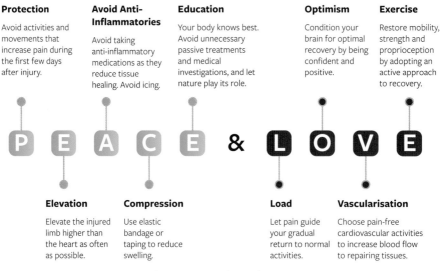

Protection

Avoid activities and movements that increase pain during the first few days after injury.

Avoid Anti-Inflammatories

Avoid taking anti-inflammatory medications as they reduce tissue healing. Avoid icing.

Education

Your body knows best. Avoid unnecessary passive treatments and medical investigations, and let nature play its role.

Optimism

Condition your brain for optimal recovery by being confident and positive.

Exercise

Restore mobility, strength and proprioception by adopting an active approach to recovery.

Elevation

Elevate the injured limb higher than the heart as often as possible.

Compression

Use elastic bandage or taping to reduce swelling.

Load

Let pain guide your gradual return to normal activities.

Vascularisation

Choose pain-free cardiovascular activities to increase blood flow to repairing tissues.

Figure 9.1 PEACE and LOVE

References

Bialosky, J.E., Bishop, M.D. and Cleland, J.A. (2010) Individual expectation: An overlooked, but pertinent, factor in the treatment of individuals experiencing musculoskeletal pain. *Physical Therapy* 90, 9, 1345–1355.

Bleakley, C.M., Glasgow, P. and MacAuley, D.C. (2012) PRICE needs updating, should we call the POLICE? *British Journal of Sports Medicine* 46, 4, 220–221.

Briet, J.P., Houwert, R.M., Hageman, M.G., Hietbrink, F., Ring, D.C. and Verleisdonk, E.J.J. (2016) Factors associated with pain intensity and physical limitations after lateral ankle sprains. *Injury* 47, 11, 2565–2569.

Chinn, L. and Hertel, J. (2010) Rehabilitation of ankle and foot injuries in athletes. *Clinics in Sports Medicine* 29, 1, 157–167.

Doherty, C., Bleakley, C., Delahunt, E. and Holden, S. (2017) Treatment and prevention of acute and recurrent ankle sprain: An overview of systematic reviews with meta-analysis. *British Journal of Sports Medicine* 51, 2, 113–125.

Dubois, B. and Esculier, J.F. (2020) Soft-tissue injuries simply need PEACE and LOVE. *British Journal of Sports Medicine* 54, 2, 72–73.

Hansrani, V., Khanbhai, M., Bhandari, S., Pillai, A. and McCollum, C.N. (2015) The role of compression in the management of soft tissue ankle injuries: A systematic review. *European Journal of Orthopaedic Surgery and Traumatology* 25, 6, 987–995.

Khan, K.M. and Scott, A. (2009) Mechanotherapy: How physical therapists' prescription of exercise promotes tissue repair. *British Journal of Sports Medicine* 43, 4, 247–252.

Lewis, J. and O'Sullivan, P. (2018) Is it time to reframe how we care for people with non-trau-matic musculoskeletal pain? *British Journal of Sports Medicine 52*, 24, 1543–1544.

Lin, I., Wiles, L., Waller, R., Goucke, R. *et al.* (2020) What does best practice care for musculoskel-etal pain look like? Eleven consistent recommendations from high-quality clinical practice guidelines: Systematic review. *British Journal of Sports Medicine 54*, 2, 79–86.

Lisowska, B., Kosson, D. and Domaracka, K. (2018) Positives and negatives of nonsteroidal anti-inflammatory drugs in bone healing: The effects of these drugs on bone repair. *Drug Design, Development and Therapy 12*, 1809–1814.

Nunes, G.S., Feldkircher, J.M., Tessarin, B.M., Bender, P.U., da Luz, C.M. and de Noronha, M. (2021) Kinesio taping does not improve ankle functional or performance in people with or without ankle injuries: Systematic review and meta-analysis. *Clinical Rehabilitation 35*, 2, 182–199.

Singh, D.P., Barani Lonbani, Z., Woodruff, M.A., Parker, T.J., Steck, R. and Peake, J.M. (2017) Effects of topical icing on inflammation, angiogenesis, revascularization, and myofiber regeneration in skeletal muscle following contusion injury. *Frontiers in Physiology 8*, 93.

Trofa, D.P., Obana, K.K., Herndon, C.L., Noticewala, M.S. *et al.* (2020) The evidence for common nonsurgical modalities in sports medicine, Part 1: Kinesio tape, sports massage therapy, and acupuncture. *JAAOS Global Research and Reviews 4*, 1, e19.00104.

Vuurberg, G., Hoorntje, A., Wink, L.M., Van Der Doelen, B.F. *et al.* (2018) Diagnosis, treatment and prevention of ankle sprains: Update of an evidence-based clinical guideline. *British Journal of Sports Medicine 52*, 15, 956–956.

Wagemans, J., Bleakley, C., Taeymans, J., Schurz, A.P. *et al.* (2022) Exercise-based rehabilita-tion reduces reinjury following acute lateral ankle sprain: A systematic review update with meta-analysis. *PLOS ONE 17*, 2, e0262023.

Wang, Z.R. and Ni, G.X. (2021) Is it time to put traditional cold therapy in rehabilitation of soft-tissue injuries out to pasture? *World Journal of Clinical Cases 9*, 17, 4116.

Ziltener, J.L., Leal, S. and Fournier, P.E. (2010) Non-steroidal anti-inflammatory drugs for ath-letes: An update. *Annals of Physical and Rehabilitation Medicine 53*, 4, 278–288.

Chapter 10

LVLA and HVLA Techniques for the Foot and Ankle

In recent years, manual therapy of the foot and ankle has gained increased attention in the orthopaedic and podiatric professions. Although healthcare professionals from various manual therapy disciplines, such as chiropractors, osteopaths and physiotherapists, have long been treating foot and ankle conditions with manipulative therapies, there is a lack of awareness among the general public regarding its usability in the treatment of lower-extremity conditions. In fact, the public perception regarding this therapy is still highly centred on back pain management. The most likely reason for this is the fact that foot manipulative techniques have not been considered an integral part of mainstream orthopaedic or podiatric practices (Menz, 1998; Hoskins *et al.*, 2006).

In clinical studies, however, manual manipulation/mobilisation of the foot and ankle has been shown to alleviate pain, immediately increase ankle range of motion, improve balance and postural control, release posterior talar glide restrictions, increase stride speed and step length, and improve weight-bearing through the foot (Dananberg, 2004; Vaillant *et al.*, 2008; Brantingham *et al.*, 2009; Shin *et al.*, 2020; Kamani *et al.*, 2021). In patients with grade I and II ankle sprains, several clinical trials have reported manual manipulation/mobilisation of the ankle to be superior compared with the RICE (rest, ice, compression and elevation) therapy and traditional exercise intervention for improving ankle mobility and function (Pellow and Brantingham, 2001; Eisenhart *et al.*, 2003; Whitman *et al.*, 2009; Gao *et al.*, 2015; Wang *et al.*, 2021). Although the clinical relevance of foot and ankle manipulation/mobilisation is still undetermined, recent systematic reviews have also concluded that these hands-on manipulative techniques appear to temporarily diminish foot pain, improve function and increase ankle range of motion, especially dorsiflexion, in patients with both acute and chronic ankle sprains (Van der Wees *et al.*, 2006; Loudon *et al.*, 2014). In addition, no detrimental effects of these techniques have been reported.

In brief, from the above discussion, it can be said that manipulation/mobilisation of the foot and ankle can alleviate pain symptoms, increase mobility of the ankle, help restore function and prevent recurrent injuries to the region. Hence, it is of critical importance for manual therapists to have professional training and adequate competency to routinely diagnose and treat lower-extremity conditions. Well-trained therapists can save many patients from chronic disability just by adding simple methods during clinical examination. For example, conditions such as fibular-related ankle equinus can easily be diagnosed with the addition of the fibular translation examination during ankle joint assessment (Dananberg, 2004).

This chapter therefore gives a general overview of foot and ankle manipulation/mobilisation – what it is, how it works and its clinical relevance in the treatment of lower-extremity conditions.

What is manipulation/mobilisation?

Manual manipulation and/or mobilisation are often described as a specialised form of manual therapy that uses drug-free, hands-on, non-invasive techniques to alleviate diverse musculoskeletal conditions. These therapies are considered relatively safe and effective when applied skilfully and appropriately. They are most commonly used to alleviate musculoskeletal pain and discomfort, reduce joint pressure and improve joint range of motion and function (Menz, 1998; Dananberg, 2004; Loudon *et al.*, 2014; Wang *et al.*, 2021).

Currently, there exists no unequivocal definition of manipulation. This is primarily owing to its colloquial function. The term 'manipulation' is too vague and frequently confused with its similar manual therapy counterparts, particularly 'mobilisation', which is still referred to as non-thrust manipulation in the literature (Whitman *et al.*, 2009; Truyols-Domínguez *et al.*, 2013). In addition, the definition of manipulation varies across various physical therapy specialities (Evans and Lucas, 2010).

From a broader classification of manipulative therapies, however, manipulation-based techniques are those that utilise a high-velocity, low-amplitude (HVLA) thrust within a joint's clinical physiological range of motion. These techniques do not allow the recipient to stop joint movement during the manoeuvre and are often accompanied by an audible cracking sound – an event usually referred to as 'cavitation' of the joint (Vernon and Mrozek, 2005;

Evans and Lucas, 2010). In contrast, mobilisation-based techniques utilise a low-velocity, low-amplitude (LVLA) approach that applies non-thrust passive motion to the joint. These techniques do not produce cavitation and the recipient is always able to stop joint movements during the manoeuvre.

How foot manipulation/mobilisation works

HVLA manipulation and joint mobilisation techniques have been shown to benefit patients with lower-extremity conditions. However, it is not yet known how these techniques exert their therapeutic effects, particularly the pain-modulatory and mobility improvement effects. To date, little research has been carried out to understand the physiological mechanisms of these techniques in the treatment of foot and ankle conditions. Menz (1998) evaluated the scientific merit of foot manipulation using a model proposed by Harris (1996) and concluded that it has some scientific basis owing to its biomechanical and neurophysiological foundation. Unfortunately, no further work has thus far been done to understand the mechanisms of foot manipulation/mobilisation.

Over the last decades, however, a significant number of mechanistic studies have been conducted on spinal HVLA manipulation and joint mobilisation. These studies concluded that the clinical effects of manipulative therapies are mediated by both biomechanical and neurophysiological mechanisms (Gevers-Montoro *et al.*, 2021; Gyer *et al.*, 2021). It has been suggested that biomechanical changes evoked following manipulation or mobilisation may trigger a chain of neural responses responsible for the observed therapeutic outcomes. In addition, the mechanical stimulus applied may influence the inflow of sensory input to the central nervous system (CNS). Until now, various neural effects of spinal manipulation have been reported in the literature, including changes in somatosensory processing, muscle-reflexogenic responses, central motor excitability, motor neuron activity, Hoffmann reflex (H-reflex) responses, sympathetic activity and central sensitisation (Bialosky *et al.*, 2009; Haavik and Murphy, 2012; Currie *et al.*, 2016; Lelic *et al.*, 2016; Randoll *et al.*, 2017; Gyer *et al.*, 2019).

It is undeniable that there are some differences between foot manipulative and spinal manipulative techniques. This is primarily due to the differences in application site as well as the way these techniques are applied. With spinal manipulation, the CNS is directly stimulated as the spine itself is included in the CNS, whereas the foot and ankle fall under the peripheral nervous system (PNS). Irrespective of these differences, however, both are actually the same treatment applied at different locations with slightly different techniques. Hence, many of the theoretical mechanisms that are applicable for spinal manipulation can also be applied to foot manipulation.

For the pain-modulatory and mobility improvement effects of foot manipulation/mobilisation, the following mechanisms may be applicable.

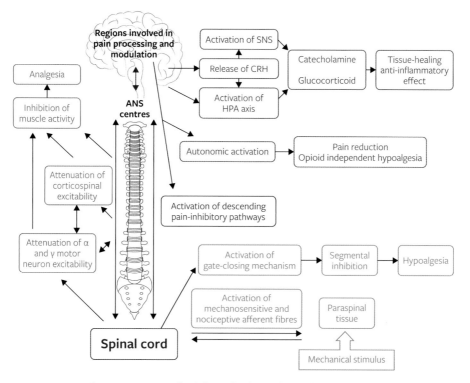

Figure 10.1 Neurophysiological effects of spinal manipulation

ANS – autonomic nervous system; CRH – corticotropin-releasing hormone; HPA axis – hypothalamic–pituitary–adrenal axis; SNS – sympathetic nervous system.

Pain gate mechanism

This theoretical mechanism is based on Melzack and Wall's (1967) gate control theory of pain. This theory proposes that nociceptive A-δ and C sensory fibres carry the pain stimuli to the dorsal horn and 'open' the substantia gelatinosa layer, while non-nociceptive A-β fibres 'close' the latter by blocking A-δ and C fibres. HVLA manipulation and joint mobilisation of the foot and ankle may influence the gate-closing mechanism by stimulating the A-β fibres, as techniques are known to alter peripheral sensory input from joint mechano-receptors (Bialosky *et al.*, 2009).

Descending inhibitory mechanism

This theorised mechanism of manipulation is based on the pain-modulatory neural circuitry. Manipulative techniques have been thought to induce non-opioid hypoalgesia by activating the descending pain modulation circuit, especially serotonin and noradrenaline pathways. Experimental studies on humans also support a nonopioid form of manipulation-induced hypoalgesic effect through activation of some type of descending inhibitory mechanism (Gyer *et al.*, 2019). However, because neural responses following manipulative therapies are reported to be dose and application-site dependent, it has been assumed that variations in mechanical parameters may activate different descending inhibitory pathways (Savva *et al.*, 2014).

Temporal summation

Temporal summation can be defined as an increased perception of pain evoked by repetitive stimulus of the same magnitude and force. Because manipulative therapies rely on force–time characteristics and can send constant nociceptive input into the dorsal horn, it is plausible to assume these therapies may induce temporal summation of pain, which also explains the mechanisms underlying hypoalgesia (Staud *et al.*, 2007; Gyer *et al.*, 2019). In fact, early experimental studies suggested that the hypoalgesic effects observed following manipulation might be regionally specific or segmental in nature. Recently, Randoll *et al.* (2017) also supported the involvement of a segmental mechanism and suggested that deep high-threshold mechanoreceptors might be responsible for HVLA-induced hypoalgesia.

Joint-gapping mechanism

The joint-gapping theory is one of the main theories that has been used for years to explain the biomechanical effects of manipulative therapies. Gapping generally denotes the separation of the joint articulation following an HVLA thrust. Joint gapping during manipulation is thought to result in an increase in joint space, stimulate nociceptive nerves that innervate the joint capsule, break up connective tissue adhesions and release the entrapped meniscoid (Evans, 2002; Cramer *et al.*, 2011).

The earlier biomechanical studies (Roston and Haines, 1947; Unsworth *et al.*, 1971) done to investigate the phenomenon of 'joint cracking' in finger metacarpophalangeal (MCP) joints showed that joint surface separation was associated with the production of cavitation and an immediate increase in radiolucent joint space. Sandoz (1976) reported that this was associated with a 5–10° increase in range of movement at the joint. In a later study, Cramer *et al.* (2000) provided further evidence in support of the joint-gapping mechanism. Using MRI scanning, the authors demonstrated an immediate increase in joint surface separation with HVLA manipulation. In this study, the average increase in gapping for the HVLA group was +1.2 mm, whereas the average change for the control group was only +0.3 mm. However, although these findings clearly support the joint-gapping theory, more work is needed to establish the true clinical significance of this theoretical mechanism.

Muscular reflexogenic mechanism

The muscular reflexogenic response is an important element of the pain–spasm–pain cycle theory of pain that has frequently been used to explain the mechanism of manipulative therapies. The muscles of the human body have some reflex responses, by means of their reflex arcs, to protect themselves from potentially harmful forces. The pain–spasm–pain cycle theory suggests that pain causes muscular hyperactivity (spasm) and muscle spasm reflexly produces pain, establishing a self-perpetuating cycle (Evans, 2002; Gyer *et al.*, 2019). HVLA manipulation and joint mobilisation techniques are thought to disrupt this pain cycle by reducing muscle activity through reflex pathways. Pickar (2002) postulated that the mechanical stimulus applied during manipulation might influence the sensory receptors to cause muscle inhibition, and suggested that afferent stimuli would target this inhibition as a reflex response. Experimental studies done to assess this theory found that manipulative therapies result in neuromuscular responses, involve spinal reflex pathways and may reduce muscle hyperactivity (Gyer *et al.*, 2019). However, it needs to be investigated whether the evoked short-latency changes in muscle response signals indicate a clinically significant outcome or merely a short-term effect.

Clinical application of foot and ankle manipulation/mobilisation

Ankle sprains and instability

Lateral ankle sprains, also known as inversion ankle sprains, occur more commonly in active people, particularly those who frequently involve themselves in sports or athletic physical activities. These sprains mostly result from forced plantarflexion/inversion movements of the ankle. In patients with ankle sprains, application of manipulative techniques at the foot and ankle region has been shown to alleviate pain, restore ankle dorsiflexion, increase stride speed and step length, and improve plantar load distribution (López-Rodríguez *et al.*, 2007; Whitman *et al.*, 2009; Truyols-Domínguez *et al.*, 2013; Shin *et al.*, 2020). A systematic review by Loudon *et al.* (2014) has also reported favourable clinical outcomes for foot manipulation and mobilisation in patients with acute, subacute and chronic ankle sprains.

However, contradictory findings are also reported in the literature (Lin *et al.*, 2010; Van Ochten *et al.*, 2014). A major complaint against manipulative therapies is that their positive clinical effects usually only last for a short time (5–7 days). On the other hand, foot manipulative techniques for ankle sprains are often applied in combination with general exercises and additional treatments. Hence, it is difficult to generalise their true clinical significance in the management of ankle sprains and ankle instability. Recently, Doherty *et al.* (2017) conducted an overview of intervention systematic reviews on ankle sprains and chronic ankle instability with a meta-analysis. After a thorough review of 46 systematic reviews, the authors concluded that early mobilisation has strong evidence for improving pain, swelling and function following an acute ankle sprain. However, they found only a moderate level of evidence supporting various manipulation techniques in the treatment of acute ankle sprains.

Ankle equinus

Ankle equinus is a condition in which the ankle joint lacks flexibility and its upward bending movement (dorsiflexion) becomes limited. Although no consensus has yet been reached in the literature on the normal degree of ankle dorsiflexion needed during the gait cycle, failure to achieve 5° of dorsiflexion with the knee extended is often considered representative of equinus. Two of the most commonly advocated treatments for this condition include daily stretching and Achilles tendon surgery (Lavery *et al.*, 2002; DeHeer, 2017).

Manual manipulation has also been known to immediately increase ankle joint dorsiflexion in patients with equinus. However, not much research has been done on this so far. Only two manipulation-based studies can be found in the literature and both were done by the same group of researchers. The first paper by Dananberg *et al.* (2000) demonstrated an immediate restoration of ankle dorsiflexion following manual manipulation of the fibula and talus. The participants in this study achieved significant dorsiflexion motion with manipulation, which was nearly twice the motion demonstrated by patients in a prior study on daily stretching. The second study (Dananberg, 2004) presented a series of cases that were successfully treated with the same manipulation techniques: (1) posterior-anterior HVLA manipulation to proximal fibular head, (2) longitudinal traction of the ankle (20–30 seconds) and (3) HVLA anterior-posterior talar thrust. All cases were able to stand and walk immediately after the manipulation session. No symptoms were reported at the three-week follow-up.

Postural control and balance

Postural control and balance can be defined as the body's ability to maintain equilibrium when exposed to a perturbation. The control of an upright posture involves a complex neuromuscular system that includes numerous sensory and motor components. Consequently, postural stability depends on the constant neuromuscular adjustments of the body to maintain the centre of gravity within the parameters of the supporting base (Dietz, 1992; Sibley *et al.*, 2015). In elderly people, these adjustments gradually deteriorate in the ageing process. As sensory inputs from the lower extremities progressively degenerate with ageing, the occurrences of falls and loss of sensory function become more and more common in the elderly (Freitas *et al.*, 2005). Hence, it has been suggested that any intervention that increases somatosensory function of the lower limbs can help improve postural control and prevent falls in the elderly (Machado *et al.*, 2017).

HVLA manipulation and joint mobilisation techniques have been known to trigger a chain of neurophysiological responses and increase the flow of sensory inputs to the brain (Gyer *et al.*, 2019). Thus, these techniques have great potential to improve postural stability and balance in the elderly. This has been demonstrated in a case series by Vaillant *et al.* (2008). The authors reported that elderly adults were compensating for functional difficulties with therapeutic manipulation of the feet and ankles. However, more research is needed into this.

Hallux limitus/rigidus

Hallux rigidus or stiff big toe is a painful condition in which degenerative arthritis affects the first metatarsophalangeal (MTP) joint. The range of motion of the MTP is reduced, particularly the extension. Hallux limitus usually denotes a less severe or early stage that precedes hallux rigidus. Until now, no conservative treatments have been found to be superior to placebo for the management of hallux rigidus. Surgery is still the treatment of choice when all empirical, traditional treatments fail. HVLA thrust manipulation and other mobilisation techniques, however, have been recommended for grade I and II hallux rigidus prior to surgery. A number of studies, including a clinical trial, case reports, case series and a Cochrane review, have supported the use of manual manipulative techniques for the treatment of hallux rigidus (Shamus *et al.*, 2004; Brantingham *et al.*, 2007; Aggarwal *et al.*, 2012; Clar *et al.*, 2014; Polzer *et al.*, 2014; Brantingham and Cassa, 2015).

Hallux valgus

Hallux valgus is a common deformity of the forefoot characterised by a medial eminence in the form of a prominent bump on the inside of the foot. The deformity usually forms when the MTP joint moves out of its normal alignment, which in turn causes the first metatarsal bone to deviate medially and the hallux to deviate laterally towards the second toe. Manual manipulation and mobilisation techniques can assist patients with hallux valgus to maintain mobility and strength in the affected MTP joint. These techniques have been shown to alleviate pain and improve function and weight-bearing both before and after surgery (Schuh *et al.*, 2009; du Plessis *et al.*, 2011; Mortka and Lisiński, 2015).

Plantar fasciitis

Plantar fasciitis is a degenerative disease of the plantar fascia. It causes stabbing pain in the heel and bottom of the foot. In patients with plantar fasciitis, the ankle joint may become compromised due to misalignment at the talus or dysfunction of the tarsal bone. As the plantar arch has ligamentous and muscular attachments with other bony structures of the foot and ankle, the changes in talus movement and tarsal function may eventually lead to motion restriction at the ankle joint and the development of plantar fasciitis symptoms. Hence, it is possible that joint mobilisation and HVLA manipulation techniques directed at the talus and talar can help address plantar fasciitis dysfunction. Several studies have suggested a trial with manipulative techniques in cases of plantar fasciitis (Polkinghorn, 1995; Dimou *et al.*, 2004; López-Rodríguez *et al.*, 2007; Schwartz and Su, 2014). Recently, Yelverton *et al.* (2019) compared three different manual therapy interventions in patients with plantar fasciitis and concluded that manual manipulation combined with cross-friction massage had a positive effect on ankle dorsiflexion, plantarflexion and pain perception.

However, the effects of joint mobilisation on plantar heel pain have been found to be controversial (Pollack *et al.*, 2018).

Red flags

It is good practice for therapists to familiarise themselves with the red flags for serious pathology in the lower extremity before pursuing manipulative interventions (WHO, 2005). Red flag symptoms help practitioners identify potentially serious pathology early and exercise sound clinical judgement to avert any potential harm to the patient. Whenever a combination of red flags in Table 10.1 is observed, manual therapists should refer patients for further clinical screening.

Table 10.1 Red flags for serious pathology in the knee, ankle and foot

Condition	Signs and symptoms
Knee fracture	History of recent trauma to the knee Intense localised swelling with effusion and ecchymosis Severe tenderness along the joint line Flexion less than 90° Patient unable to walk more than four weight-bearing steps
Compartment syndrome	History of blunt trauma Cumulative trauma Overuse Intense, persistent pain and firmness to anterior shin compartment Reduced pulse Paraesthesia Pain with toe dorsiflexion Intense pain associated with stretch on affected muscles
Extensor mechanism disruption	Quadriceps or patella tendon rupture Superior translation of the patella
Fractures	Trauma from a motor vehicle accident, blunt force to the ankle or a fall Inflammation on affected leg with concomitant pain Relentless synovitis Involved tissues feel sore and are highly sensitive Difficulty walking more than four weight-bearing steps

Deep vein thrombosis	Recent surgery, period of limited mobility, pregnancy or malignancy
	Hot, erythemic and very tender calf
	Fever and malaise
	Positive cc
	Pain exaggerated with use of the extremity (i.e. walking or standing) and diminished with rest
Septic arthritis	Fever and chills accompanied by consistent pain
	History of bacterial infection
	Recent invasive medical intervention (e.g. surgery or injection)
	Open wound
	Joint inflammation with no history of trauma
	General malaise or loss of appetite
	Compromised immunity
Cancer	Chronic pain with no history of trauma
	History of malignancy
	Weight loss with no clear explanation
	General malaise with or without fever and weakness
	Presence of swelling or unexplained presence of tumours and deformity

Sources: Boissonnault (2005); Stephenson (2013); Magee (2014); Wise (2015)

Special tests

Table 10.2 Special tests for knee, ankle and foot dysfunction

Test	Procedure	Positive sign	Interpretation	Test statistics
Lachman/ Trillat/ Ritchie test	In this one-plane test, the patient assumes a supine posture. The patient's foot is stabilised between the therapist's thigh and the couch. With the therapist's outside hand stabilising the femur, he/she applies gentle force pulling the tibia forward, with the intent of generating anterior translation.	Excessive anterior excursion of the tibia on the femur accompanied by a soft or absent joint end-feel Diminishing of the normal slope of the infrapatellar tendon	Anterior cruciate ligament injury May also indicate injury to the posterior oblique ligament or arcuate-popliteus complex	Specificity: 0.91 Sensitivity: 0.86

Test	Procedure	Positive sign	Interpretation	Test statistics
Posterior drawer test	With the patient lying supine, the hip and knee are flexed at 45° and 90° respectively, with the tibia in neutral rotation. The therapist pushes backwards on the tibia after stabilising the patient's foot.	Posterior movement of the tibia relative to the femur	Posterior cruciate ligament laxity	Specificity: 0.99 Sensitivity: 0.90
Abduction/valgus stress test	In this one-plane medial instability assessment, the therapist pushes the patient's knee medially (valgus stress) while stabilising the ankle in slight lateral rotation. The knee is typically in full extension and 30° flexion. The test thigh may be rested on the table to help the patient relax.	Medial collateral ligament laxity on application of valgus stress	Injury to posterior and medial cruciate ligaments	Specificity: not reported Sensitivity: 0.91
McMurray's test	The patient assumes a supine position with the knee in full flexion. The therapist rotates the tibia medially while extending the knee. The therapist repeatedly changes the amount of flexion while applying medial rotation and then extension to the tibia to test the complete posterior aspect of the meniscus (i.e. posterior horn to middle segment).	A snap or click accompanied by pain	Loose meniscal fragment	Specificity: 0.93 Sensitivity: 0.59
Talar tilt test	The patient lies supine or on the side with the foot relaxed. The normal side is tested first to establish a point of comparison. With the therapist holding the foot at 90°, the talus is tilted from side to side into inversion and eversion.	An increased talar tilt or joint laxity when compared with the normal side	Torn calcaneofibular ligament	Specificity: 0.74 Sensitivity: 0.52

Thompson's/ Simmonds' test	The patient assumes a prone position or kneels on a chair with the feet hanging over the edge of the chair. With the patient relaxed, the therapist squeezes the calf muscles.	Absence of plantarflexion when the calf muscle is squeezed	Achilles tendon rupture	Specificity: 0.93 Sensitivity: 0.96
Anterior drawer test	With the patient lying prone, the ankle in a neutral position and the foot in 20° of plantarflexion, the therapist applies an anteriorly directed force to the calcaneus. This may also be done by pushing backwards on the tibia.	Increased anterior translation compared to the normal side	Anterior talocrural joint laxity	Specificity: 0.38 Sensitivity: 0.74
Kleiger test (external rotation stress test)	The patient is seated, while flexing the knee at 90°. The therapist stabilises the leg with one hand and applies a passive lateral rotational stress externally to the affected foot and ankle.	Significant pain at the anterolateral part of the distal tibiofibular syndesmosis	Syndesmotic injury Deltoid ligament injury	Specificity: 0.85 Sensitivity: 0.20

Sources: Malanga et al. (2003); Boissonnault (2005); Ostrowski (2006); Manske and Prohaska (2008); Hattam and Smeatham (2010); de César et al. (2011); Croy et al. (2013); Douglas et al. (2013); Schwieterman et al. (2013); Magee (2014); Slaughter et al. (2014); Wise (2015)

Osteopathic articulation and mobilisation (LVLA) techniques for the foot and ankle

Talonavicular joint

- Facing away from the patient, fix the foot in a neutral position with your index finger posterior to the navicular.

- Grasp the foot with the other hand, aligning index fingers.

- With straight arms, use your bodyweight to articulate through the talonavicular joint.

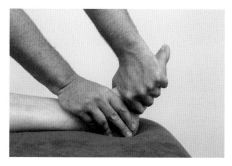

Naviculocuneiform joint

- Facing away from the patient, fix the foot in a neutral position with your index finger on the navicular.

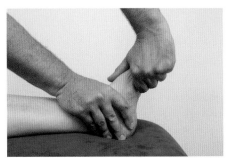

- Grasp the foot with the other hand, covering the cuneiform and metatarsals.

- With straight arms, use your bodyweight to articulate through the naviculocuneiform joint.

Tarsometatarsal joint

- Facing away from the patient, fix the foot in a neutral position, covering the navicular and medial cuneiform.

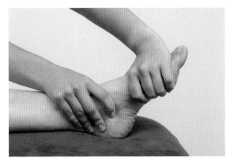

- Grasp the foot with the other hand, covering the first metatarsal.

- With straight arms, use your bodyweight to articulate through the tarsometatarsal joint.

Medial border

- Standing at the end of the plinth, fix around the talus and navicular.

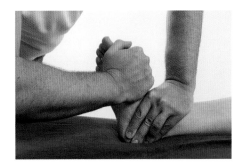

- With the other hand, grasp around the medial aspect of the foot to articulate the medial cuneiform on the navicular.

Prone medial border

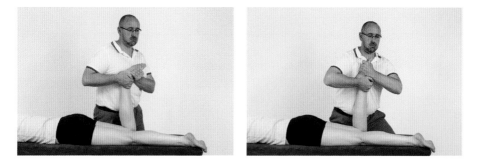

- Stand at the side of the plinth, with the patient's nearest leg flexed to 90° at the knee.

- Fix around the medial ankle.

- Grasp around the navicular and medial cuneiform and use a scooping motion to articulate the talonavicular joint.

- Slide the hands along to articulate the naviculocuneiform and cuneiform metatarsal joints.

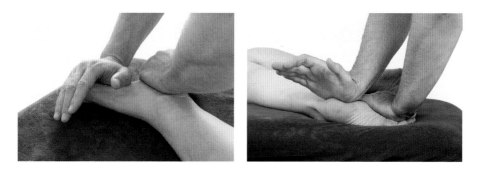

- Stand at the end of the plinth, with the patient lying on the affected side with the knee bent.

- Use a cross-hand technique on the calcaneus to fix the foot into dorsiflexion.

- With the other hand, invert the foot by applying pressure over the navicular.

- Adjust the pressure between the hands to articulate the subtalar joint.

Anterior glide

- Stand at the lower side of the plinth in a split stance.

- Cup under the calcaneus with one hand and fix across the distal tibia and fibula with the other.

- With straight arms, rock on to your back foot to initiate an anterior glide of the talus against the tibia and fibula.

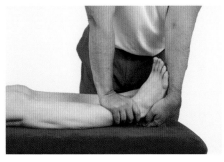

Posterior glide

- Stand at the lower side of the plinth in a split stance.

- Stabilise the foot into the plinth in a neutral position with the lower hand.

- Grasp around the tibia and fibula with the other hand.

- Drop your weight through the lower hand to glide the talus posterior to the tibia and fibula.

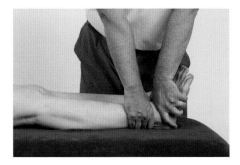

Plantarflexion

- Stabilise the patient's leg on the plinth.

- Cup the calcaneus with sole of the foot resting on your forearm.

- Scoop the calcaneus posteriorly to articulate the talocrural joint into plantarflexion.

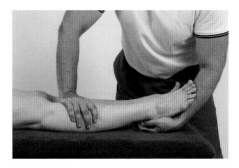

Traction to talocrural joint supine

- Place the patient's knee over your flexed knee on the plinth.

- With your elbow supported against your knee, fix the lower hand behind the calcaneus.

- The upper hand dorsiflexes the foot and drives downward towards the plinth.

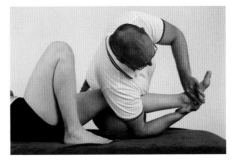

Adaptive traction to talocrural joint supine

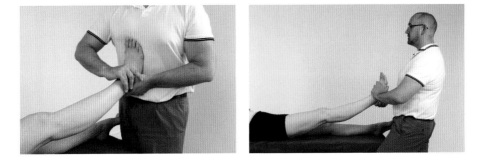

- Standing at the end of the plinth, cup under the calcaneus with one hand and around the talus with the other.

- With a split stance and keeping your arms close to your body, shift your weight on to your back leg to create traction at the talocrural joint.

Talocrural prone shift

- Stand at the end of the plinth medial to the leg with the patient's foot off the end.

- Hook under the tibia with one hand and place the corresponding hand webbed around the posterior aspect of the calcaneus.

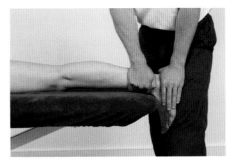

- With a split stance, drop your weight through the calcaneus towards the floor to glide the talus forward on the tibia.

Talocrural shearing

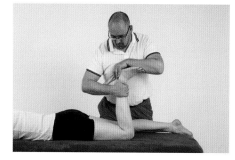

- Stand at the side of the plinth, with the patient prone.

- Flex the knee and foot to 90°.

- Grasp around the anterior aspect of the ankle with the other hand on the posterior aspect of the calcaneus.

- Apply opposing forces with the arms to create shearing at the talocrural joint.

Subtalar inversion/eversion

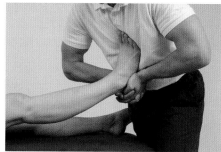

- Standing at the end of the plinth, brace the foot against the lower sternum. Lean forward to dorsiflex the foot.

- Interlock the fingers and cup around the calcaneus.

- In this fixed position, rotate your torso to create inversion and eversion of the subtalar joint.

Anterior mobilisation talocrural

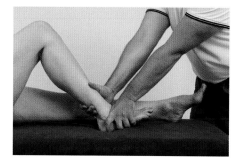

- Stand at the foot of the plinth in a split stance.

- Flex the patient's knee and foot to 90° angles.

- Stabilise the foot around the talus with one hand.

- The corresponding hand grips the lower leg around the tibia.

- With straight arms, shift your weight on to the back leg to drive the tibia and fibula anterior to the talus.

Posterior mobilisation

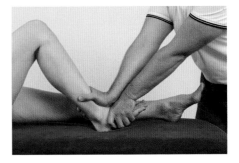

- Stand at the foot of the plinth in a split stance.

- Flex the patient's knee and foot to 90° angles.

- Stabilise the foot around the talus with one hand.

- The corresponding hand grips anteriorly around the tibia.

- With straight arms, shift your weight on to the front leg to drive the tibia and fibula posterior to the talus.

Calcaneus–cuboid

- Stand at the side of the plinth, facing away from the patient.

- Cup under the calcaneus on the medial side of the leg with the forearm resting on the plinth.

- With the thenar eminence and fingers of the corresponding hand, grip around the cuboid and fourth and fifth metatarsals.

- With straight arms, shift your weight on to the front and back legs to mobilise the cuboid on the calcaneus.

Cuboid-metatarsals

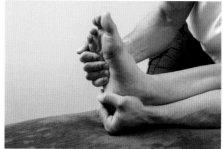

- Stand at the side of the plinth, facing away from the patient.

- Cup under the calcaneus and cuboid on the medial side of the leg with the forearm resting on the plinth.

- With the thenar eminence and fingers of the corresponding hand, grip around the fourth and fifth metatarsals.

- With straight arms, shift your weight on to the front and back legs to mobilise the metatarsals on the cuboid.

Lateral border

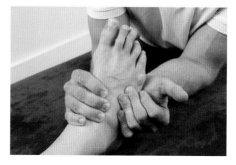

- Stand at the foot of the plinth.

- Grasp the medial aspect of the foot, keeping it in a neutral position with your thumb fixed on the cuboid.

- Hold the fourth and fifth metatarsals between the thenar eminence and fingers.

- Articulate the metatarsals against the fixed cuboid.

Cuneiform

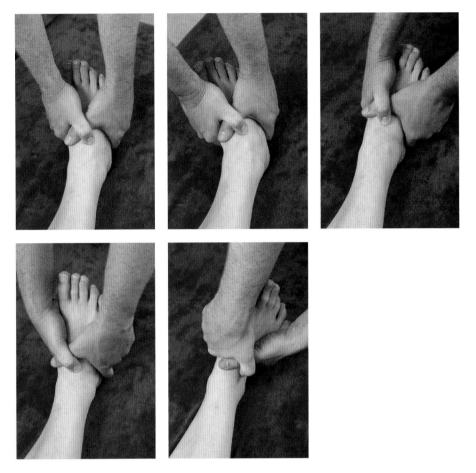

- Stand at the foot of the plinth.

- Grasp around the foot with both hands, crossing the thumbs on the dorsum of the foot over the targeted cuneiform.

- Articulate the targeted joint in an imaginary figure-of-eight motion as demonstrated in the photos.

Hallux traction

- Stand at the foot of the plinth. Support the foot with one hand around the metatarsals.

- Grasp the metatarsophalangeal joint of the hallux, with the thumb over the joint.

- Articulate the joint by applying traction and circumduction forces.

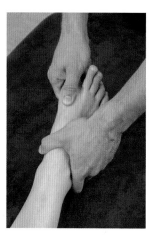

Toe traction

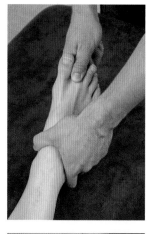 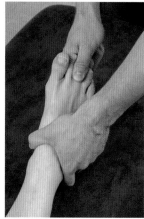 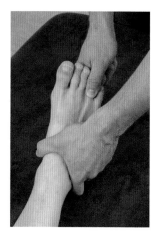

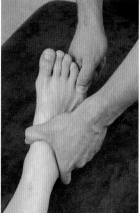

- Stand at the end of the plinth. Support the foot with one hand around the metatarsals.

- Grasp the metatarsophalangeal joint with the thumb over the joint.

- Articulate the joint by applying traction and circumduction forces.

Cuboid prone

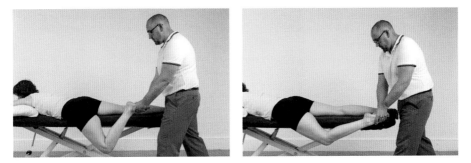

- Stand at the lower corner of the plinth.

- With the patient's knee off the table, grasp the foot with both hands, crossing your thumbs over the plantar aspect of the cuboid.

- Articulate from a dorsiflexed to a plantarflexed position by extending the hip and the knee, driving through the tibia.

- Maintain abduction, inversion and compression with the fingers.

Osteopathic and chiropractic (HVLA) techniques for the foot and ankle

Tibiotalar manipulation

- Have the patient in a supine position, with hip and knee flexed between 45° and 90°.

- For comfort, place a towel under the patient's tibia and foot.

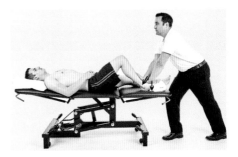

- Position yourself at the foot of the table with an asymmetrical stance.

- Your right hand contacts the medial aspect of the calcaneus.

- Your left hand contacts the midfoot. Your first MCP contacts the navicular and supinates the foot.

- Ask the patient to inhale and exhale.

- At the end of the exhalation, engage the barrier by increasing tension through both hands.

Supine tibiotalar manipulation

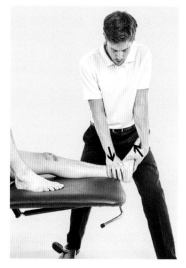

- The patient is in supine position with the foot just off the table as shown.

- For the patient's comfort, place a towel underneath the lower leg.

- Stand at the foot of the table with an asymmetrical stance, facing the foot as shown.

- Place your right hand, with a broad contact between the thumb and index finger, just inferior to the malleoli.

- Your left hand contacts around the plantar aspect of the foot with the fingers facing towards the floor.

- Ask the patient to inhale and exhale.

- At the end of exhalation, engage the barrier.

- Once the barrier is engaged, manipulate the joint by creating medial to lateral (ML) force with your left hand.

- The stabilising hand does just that. There is no need to thrust with this hand.

Prone tibiotalar manipulation

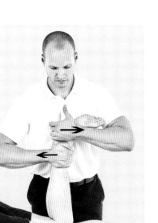

- The patient is in the prone position.

- Stand to the side of the table, on the side you will be manipulating.

- Flex the knee to 90°.

- Place your right hand around the distal tibia and fibula as close to the tibiotalar joint as possible.

- Place your left hand around the posterior aspect of the calcaneus.

- Ask the patient to inhale and exhale.

- Halfway through the exhalation phase, begin to engage the barrier by pulling your hands apart and towards your sternum.

- To manipulate the joint, perform a rapid pulling-apart motion of the hands while bringing your elbows to your side.

Crouching subtalar manipulation

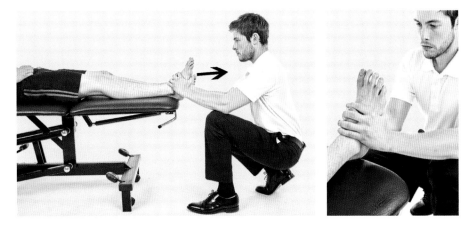

- The patient is in supine position.

- Stand at the foot of the table, facing the patient, then crouch to be level with the table.

- Use an asymmetrical squat posture.

- Both fifth metacarpals are interlinked and cover the trochlea of the talus.

- With your lateral hand, take up the skin slack and create a lateral draw towards the fifth tarsal.

- Bring both thumbs under the plantar aspect of the foot and contact under the distal portion of the calcaneus.

- Create internal or external rotation of the limb to lock out the hip.

- Ask the patient to inhale and exhale.

- On exhalation, engage the barrier and perform the manipulation by pulling through your elbows.

Side-lying subtalar

- Have the patient lie on the side of the foot you wish to manipulate with the knee bent at 90°.

- For the patient's comfort, place a towel underneath the lower leg.

- Adopt an asymmetrical stance.

- Adjust the height of the table to allow you to contact the patient's foot with your arms almost straight.

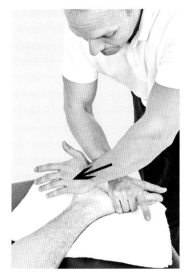

- Place your left hand, with a broad contact between the thumb and index finger, over the distal lower leg, as close to the talocrural joint as possible.

- Place your right hand over the posterior to medial (PM) aspect of the calcaneus.

- Ask the patient to inhale and exhale; at the end of exhalation, the barrier should be engaged.

- Perform an ML manipulation with your right hand down towards the floor.

Side-lying subtalar manipulation

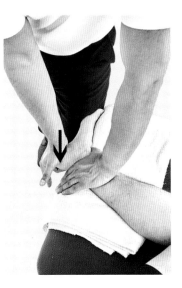

- Have the patient lie on the side of the foot you wish to manipulate, with the knee bent at 90°; the foot should be hanging just over the side of the table.

- Stand at the side of the table, facing towards it.

- Adjust the height of the table to allow you to contact the patient's foot with arms almost straight.

- Place your left hand, with a broad contact between the thumb and index finger, over the distal lower leg, as close to the talocrural joint as possible.

- Place your right hand over the PM aspect of the calcaneus.

- Ask the patient to inhale and exhale; at the end of exhalation, the barrier should be engaged.

- Perform an ML manipulation with your right hand down towards the floor.

Standing subtalar manipulation

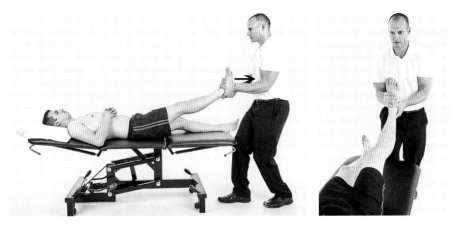

- The patient is in supine position.

- Stand at the foot of the table, facing the patient, with an asymmetrical stance.

- Your left hand contacts the calcaneus and your right hand contacts the trochlea of the talus with your fifth metacarpal.

- Use the thumb of your right hand to create a slight dorsiflexion of the ankle.

- Create internal or external rotation of the limb to lock out the hip and decrease the movement potential of the joint.

- Ask the patient to inhale and exhale.

- At the end of the exhalation phase, engage the barrier and manipulate the joint.

- The manipulation is achieved by pulling your elbows sharply towards you and leaning on to your back foot to use your body weight.

Prone talocalcaneal manipulation

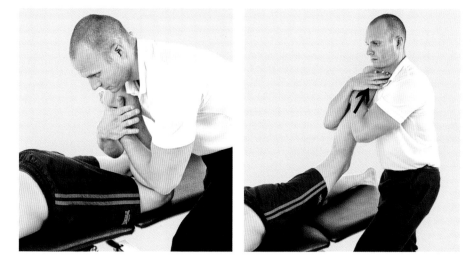

- Have the patient in a prone position, with the ankle to be manipulated closest to the side of the couch. (The photos show the left ankle being manipulated so the technique is performed on your right-hand side.)

- Flex the knee up to 90° to allow you to take hold of the calcaneus between the thumb and forefinger of both hands.

- Your hands will fit tightly against the posterior aspect of the calcaneus.

- Rest the anterior aspect of the foot over your shoulder.

- As you stand up, move posteriorly and obliquely to bring on slight traction to the talocalcaneal joint.

- Ask the patient to inhale and exhale.

- Halfway through the exhalation phase, engage the barrier.

- The manipulation is given through your legs; your arms are there to stabilise the joint. When you reach the barrier of the joint, stand up, performing the manipulation in a superior to oblique (SO) direction.

Talocalcaneal manipulation

- Ask the patient to lie in the supine position.

- Stand at the foot of the table, facing towards the patient, with an asymmetrical stance.

- With your fingers pointing towards the floor, your left hand contacts the calcaneus on both sides as shown.

- Your left hand is over the medial aspect of the calcaneonavicular joint.

- Your right hand is in contact with the distal fibula so that your fingers rest above the fingers of the hand gripping the calcaneus.

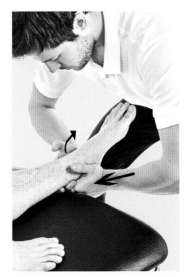

- Ask the patient to inhale and exhale, and engage the barrier.

- Once the barrier is engaged, perform the manipulation in a movement from ML with your right hand.

- At the same time, your left hand contacting the distal fibula is manipulated posterior to anterior (PA).

Talonavicular manipulation

- Ask the patient to lie in the supine position.

- Adopt an asymmetrical stance on the ipsilateral side of the table, facing the foot you are manipulating.

- Both arms need to be near full extension at the elbow.

- With your left hand, place your index finger on the navicular tuberosity.

- Stabilise the patient's distal tibia/fibula with a broad-based contact, using your right hand as shown.

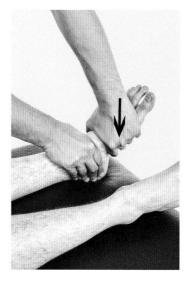

- Ask the patient to inhale and exhale.

- At the end of exhalation, engage the barrier by pronating the foot via the navicular with slight plantarflexion.

- Once you have engaged the barrier, perform the manipulation with a short, sharp movement incorporating the pronation and slight plantarflexion.

Midfoot manipulation (talonavicular and navicular cuneiforms)

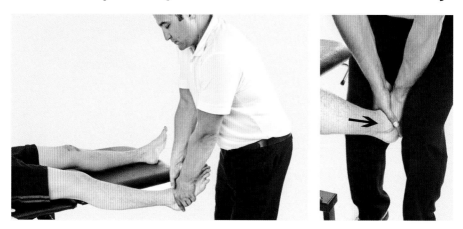

- The patient is in the supine position.

- Approach the bench and hold the working foot in both hands.

- Stand at the foot of the table, facing the patient, using an asymmetrical stance.

- With the fifth metacarpal of your right hand, cover the trochlea of the talus.

- Your left hand holds on to the calcaneus.

- Create internal or external rotation of the limb to lock out the hip.

- Ask the patient to inhale and exhale.

- On the exhalation phase, engage the barrier and perform the manipulation by pulling through your elbows.

Navicular manipulation

- The patient is in the supine position.

- Stand on the ipsilateral side of the table to the side you are manipulating.

- With the knee and hip flexed to 90°, the foot is roughly level with the middle of your sternum.

- Your left hand contacts over the talocrural joint with all five fingers, resting the palm of your hand over the medial aspect of the patient's calcaneus.

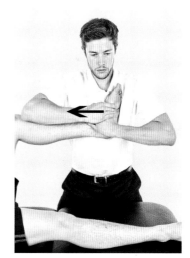

- Your right hand is over the medial aspect of the foot so that the first, fourth and fifth fingers are relaxed and resting over the plantar aspect.

- The contact point for the manipulation is the proximal interphalangeal joint of the third finger. Ensure that when positioning the contact hand, this joint is in contact with the navicular tuberosity.

- To complete set-up, ensure that the forearm of the contact hand is parallel and resting lightly on the patient's shin.

- Ask the patient to inhale and exhale. At the end of exhalation, engage the barrier.

- To manipulate the joint, perform a rapid pulling-apart motion of the hands while bringing your elbows to your side.

Prone cuboid manipulation

- The patient lies prone, slightly off centre and closer to the side of the table you are standing near.

- Hold the foot with both hands and adopt an asymmetrical stance.

- Bring the affected foot off the table, allowing knee and hip flexion.

- Contact over the lateral border of the foot and palpate the cuboid.

- Your left thumb covers the posterior aspect of the cuboid; support your thumb with the other thumb crossed over.

- Ask the patient to inhale and exhale.

- Towards the end of the exhalation phase, engage the barrier.

- Keeping your body weight directly over the points of contact, manipulate downward and slightly oblique.

- The manipulation occurs from a slight extension of both arms and a small forward movement through your legs.

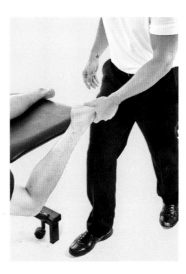

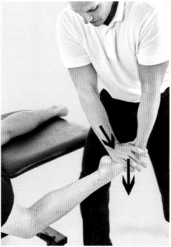

Phalangeal manipulation

- The patient is in the supine position.

- Adopt an asymmetrical stance.

- Your right hand stabilises over the talonavicular joint.

- Your left hand contacts the toe between the thumb and palm.

- Ask the patient to inhale and exhale. At the end of exhalation, engage the barrier.

- Perform the manipulation by pulling towards you.

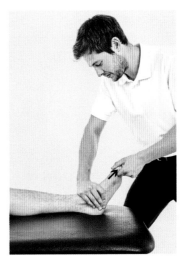

Cuneiform manipulation in supine

- The patient is lying in the supine position.

- Maintain an asymmetrical stance position as shown.

- Clasp your hands together on the anterior and posterior aspect of the target cuneiform as shown.

- Ask the patient to inhale and then slowly exhale.

- As the patient starts to exhale, begin to build the barrier inferiorly.

- At the engagement of the barrier, apply the manipulation inferiorly.

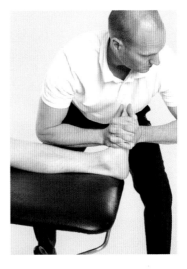

Tibiotalar manipulation in supine

- The patient is lying in the supine position.

- Adopt an asymmetrical stance as shown.

- Using both hands, contact just below the medial and lateral malleolus.

- The pads of your thumbs should make contact with the trochlea of the talus.

- Ask the patient to inhale and then slowly exhale.

- As the patient starts to exhale, stabilise the target by clasping your hands together as shown and create traction.

- At the end of exhalation, apply the manipulation towards you.

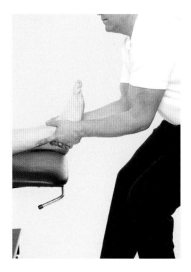

Metatarsal head manipulation

- The patient is lying in the supine position.

- Adopt an asymmetrical stance.

- Interlace your fingers over the target metatarsal head.

- Your thumbs can add plantar or dorsiflexion as needed.

- Ask the patient to inhale and then slowly exhale.

- At the end of exhalation, apply the manipulation towards you.

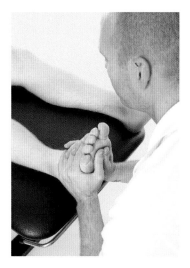

Talus manipulation in supine

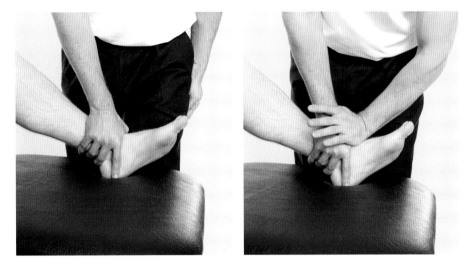

- The patient is lying in the supine position with their knee in flexion.

- Adopt an asymmetrical stance as shown.

- Your hand stabilises the medial and lateral malleolus.

- Your other hand contacts the trochlea of the talus down towards the table.

- Ask the patient to inhale and then slowly exhale.

- As the patient starts to exhale, add your pressure in an oblique direction to engage the barrier.

- At the end of exhalation, the barrier should be engaged; perform the manipulation down towards the table.

Navicular manipulation in supine

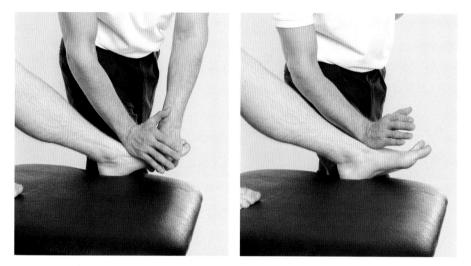

- The patient is lying in the supine position with their knee in flexion and calcaneus in contact with the table.

- Adopt an asymmetrical stance as shown.

- Your left thumb makes contact on the superior aspect of the navicular reinforced by the pisiform of your right hand.

- Ask the patient to inhale and then slowly exhale.

- As the patient starts to exhale, add your pressure in an oblique direction to engage the barrier.

- At the end of exhalation, the barrier should be engaged; perform the manipulation downwards and slightly oblique to the table.

Medial cuneiform and first metatarsal manipulation

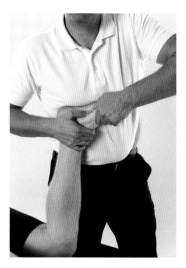

- The patient is lying in the prone position with their knee in flexion, with the plantar aspect of the foot held as shown against your abdomen.

- Adopt an asymmetrical stance as shown.

- Your thenar eminence stabilises the medial aspect of the foot, while your thumb applies static pressure to the cuneiform.

- Ask the patient to inhale and then slowly exhale.

- As the patient starts to exhale, you increase inversion of the first metatarsal.

- At the end of exhalation, the barrier should be engaged; perform the manipulation upwards.

Navicular manipulation in supine with extended leg

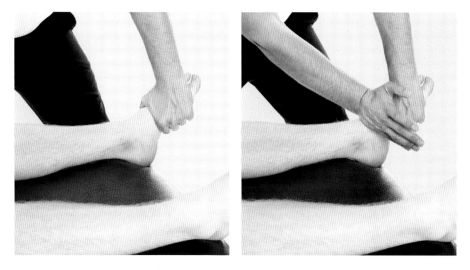

- The patient is lying in the supine position with their knee in full extension for stability.

- Adopt an asymmetrical stance as shown.

- Locate and hold the navicular as shown.

- Your other hand, via the pisiform, rests on top of your hand.

- Ask the patient to inhale and then slowly exhale.

- As the patient starts to exhale, begin to build the barrier.

- At the end of exhalation, the barrier should be engaged; perform the manipulation inferior and oblique towards the floor.

Navicular manipulation in supine position with knee in flexion

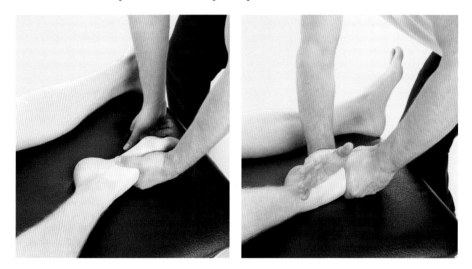

- The patient is lying in the supine position with their knee in flexion and the hip externally rotated.

- Adopt an asymmetrical stance.

- Locate and hold the first metatarsal as shown.

- Your other hand, via the pisiform, contacts the navicular tubercle as shown.

- Ask the patient to inhale and then slowly exhale.

- As the patient starts to exhale, begin to build the barrier by rotating the first metatarsal towards you and pushing the navicular obliquely towards the table.

- At the end of exhalation, the barrier should be engaged; perform the manipulation towards the table via the contact hand on the navicular.

Proximal first metatarsal with knee flexion

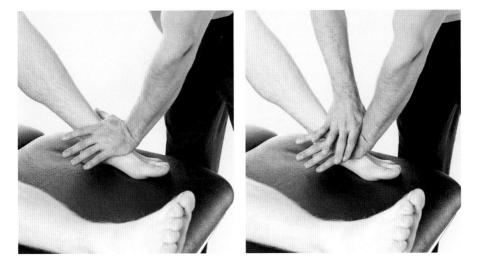

- The patient is lying in the supine position with their knee in flexion.

- Adopt an asymmetrical stance.

- Locate the proximal head of the first metatarsal and make contact via the pisiform as shown.

- Using the web of your free hand, make contact on your hand as shown.

- Ask the patient to inhale and then slowly exhale.

- As the patient starts to exhale, begin to build the barrier by adding downward pressure through your top hand.

- At the end of exhalation, the barrier should be engaged; perform the manipulation towards the table via the contact hand on the navicular.

Hallux manipulation

- The patient is lying in the supine position with their knee in extension.

- Take hold of the hallux with one hand as shown.

- With your other hand, contact the joint line of the first metatarsal.

- Ask the patient to inhale and then slowly exhale.

- As the patient starts to exhale, begin to build the barrier in the directions shown.

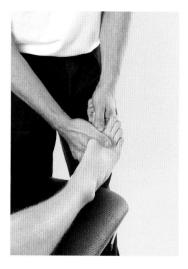

- At the end of exhalation, the barrier should be engaged; perform the manipulation in the transverse direction along the line of the first metatarsal.

Calcaneus manipulation in prone

- The patient is lying in the prone position.

- Maintain an asymmetrical stance.

- With one hand, stabilise the lower leg while the other hand contacts with the posterior aspect of the calcaneus as shown.

- Ask the patient to inhale and then slowly exhale.

- As the patient starts to exhale, begin to build the barrier by applying pressure down towards the floor.

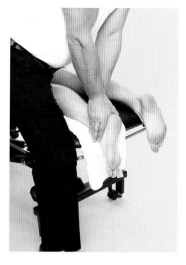

- At the end of exhalation, the barrier should be engaged; perform the manipulation towards the floor.

Tibiotalar manipulation

- The patient is lying in the prone position.

- Maintain an asymmetrical stance.

- With one hand, stabilise the lower leg while the other hand contacts with the posterior aspect of the calcaneus as shown.

- Ask the patient to inhale and then slowly exhale.

- At the end of exhalation, the barrier should be engaged; perform the manipulation by pulling the tibia towards you while simultaneously pushing the calcaneus down.

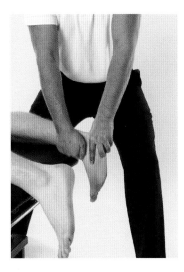

Talocrural manipulation

- The patient is lying in the prone position.

- Maintain an asymmetrical stance.

- Make contact on the trochlea of the talus and calcaneus as shown.

- Ask the patient to inhale and then slowly exhale.

- As the patient starts to exhale, begin to build the barrier by applying traction towards you.

- At the end of exhalation, the barrier should be engaged; perform the manipulation by pulling the talus and calcaneus towards you.

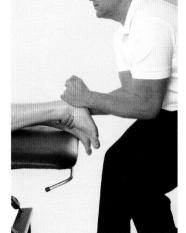

Cuneiform manipulation

- The patient is lying in the supine position.

- Maintain an asymmetrical stance.

- Make contact on the posterior aspect of the calcaneus while making contact on the target cuneiform as shown.

- Ask the patient to inhale and then slowly exhale.

- As the patient starts to exhale, begin to build the barrier by stabilising the calcaneus and pushing the cuneiform inferiorly.

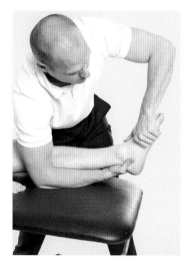

- Once you have engaged the barrier, create a short, fast manipulation cavitating the joint.

Cuboid manipulation

- The patient is lying in the prone position.

- Maintain an asymmetrical stance.

- Make contact on the posterior aspect of the cuboid with your thumb, which is reinforced by the pisiform as shown.

- Ask the patient to inhale and then slowly exhale.

- As the patient starts to exhale, you begin to build the barrier by plantar-flexing the foot while adding down-wards pressure.

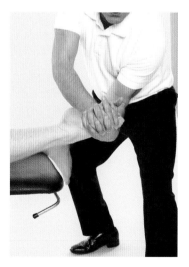

- Once the barrier is engaged, perform the manipulation via the pisiform contact laterally and towards the floor.

Cuboid manipulation

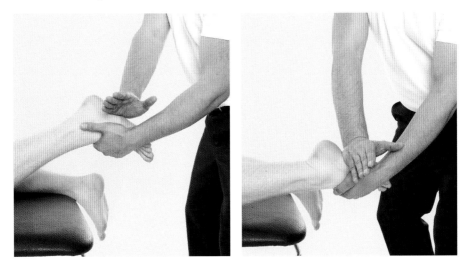

- The patient is lying in the prone position.

- Maintain an asymmetrical stance position.

- Your left hand controls the dorsal aspect of the foot while the ulnar border of your right hand makes contact on the posterior aspect of the cuboid.

- Ask the patient to inhale and then slowly exhale.

- As the patient starts to exhale, begin to build the barrier by plantar-flexing the foot while adding downward pressure.

- Once the barrier is engaged, perform the manipulation via the pisiform contact towards the floor.

Adaptive cuboid manipulation

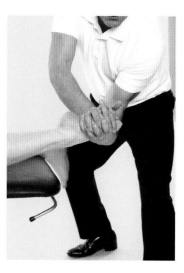

- The patient is lying in the prone position.

- Maintain an asymmetrical stance.

- Using both hands, contact the dorsal aspect of the target foot and cross your thumbs over the posterior aspect of the target cuboid as shown.

- Ask the patient to inhale and then slowly exhale.

- As the patient starts to exhale, begin to build the barrier by plantarflexing the foot while adding downward pressure through your thumbs.

- Once the barrier is engaged, perform the manipulation laterally and inferiorly.

References

Aggarwal, A., Kumar, S. and Kumar, R. (2012) Therapeutic management of the hallux rigidus. *Rehabilitation Research and Practice 2012*, 479046.

Bialosky, J.E., Bishop, M.D., Price, D.D., Robinson, M.E. and George, S.Z. (2009) The mechanisms of manual therapy in the treatment of musculoskeletal pain: A comprehensive model. *Manual Therapy 14*, 5, 531–538.

Boissonnault, W.G. (2005) *Primary Care for the Physical Therapist*. Elsevier Saunders.

Brantingham, J.W. and Cassa, T.K. (2015) Manipulative and multimodal therapies in the treatment of osteoarthritis of the great toe: A case series. *Journal of Chiropractic Medicine 14*, 4, 270–278.

Brantingham, J.W., Chang, M.N., Gendreau, D.F. and Price, J.L. (2007) The effect of chiropractic adjusting, exercises and modalities on a 32-year-old professional male golfer with hallux rigidus. *Clinical Chiropractic 10*, 2, 91–96.

Brantingham, J.W., Globe, G., Pollard, H., Hicks, M., Korporaal, C. and Hoskins, W. (2009) Manipulative therapy for lower extremity conditions: Expansion of literature review. *Journal of Manipulative and Physiological Therapeutics 32*, 1, 53–71.

Clar, C., Tsertsvadze, A., Hundt, G.L., Clarke, A. and Sutcliffe, P. (2014) Clinical effectiveness of manual therapy for the management of musculoskeletal and non-musculoskeletal conditions: Systematic review and update of UK evidence report. *Chiropractic and Manual Therapies 22*, 1, 1–34.

Cramer, G.D., Ross, K., Pocius, J., Cantu, J.A. *et al.* (2011) Evaluating the relationship among cavitation, zygapophyseal joint gapping, and spinal manipulation: An exploratory case series. *Journal of Manipulative and Physiological Therapeutics* 34, 1, 2–14.

Cramer, G.D., Tuck, N.R., Knudsen, J.T., Fonda, S.D. *et al.* (2000) Effects of side-posture positioning and side-posture adjusting on the lumbar zygapophysial joints as evaluated by magnetic resonance imaging: A before and after study with randomization. *Journal of Manipulative and Physiological Therapeutics* 23, 6, 380–394.

Croy, T., Koppenhaver, S., Saliba, S. and Hertel, J. (2013) Anterior talocrural joint laxity: Diagnostic accuracy of the anterior drawer test of the ankle. *Journal of Orthopaedic and Sports Physical Therapy* 43, 12, 911–919.

Currie, S.J., Myers, C.A., Durso, C., Enebo, B.A. and Davidson, B.S. (2016) The neuromuscular response to spinal manipulation in the presence of pain. *Journal of Manipulative and Physiological Therapeutics* 39, 4, 288–293.

Dananberg, H.J. (2004) Manipulation of the ankle as a method of treatment for ankle and foot pain. *Journal of the American Podiatric Medical Association* 94, 4, 395–399.

Dananberg, H.J., Shearstone, J. and Guillano, M. (2000) Manipulation method for the treatment of ankle equinus. *Journal of the American Podiatric Medical Association* 90, 8, 385–389.

de César, P.C., Ávila, E.M. and de Abreu, M.R. (2011) Comparison of magnetic resonance imaging to physical examination for syndesmotic injury after lateral ankle sprain. *Foot and Ankle International* 32, 12, 1110–1114.

DeHeer, P.A. (2017) Equinus and lengthening techniques. *Clinics in Podiatric Medicine and Surgery* 34, 2, 207–227.

Dietz, V. (1992) Human neuronal control of automatic functional movements: Interaction between central programs and afferent input. *Physiological Reviews* 72, 1, 33–69.

Dimou, E.S., Brantingham, J.W. and Wood, T. (2004) A randomized, controlled trial (with blinded observer) of chiropractic manipulation and Achilles stretching vs. orthotics for the treatment of plantar fasciitis. *Journal of the American Chiropractic Association* 41, 9, 32–42.

Doherty, C., Bleakley, C., Delahunt, E. and Holden, S. (2017) Treatment and prevention of acute and recurrent ankle sprain: An overview of systematic reviews with meta-analysis. *British Journal of Sports Medicine* 51, 2, 113–125.

Douglas, G., Nicol, F. and Robertson, C. (eds) (2013) *Macleod's Clinical Examination*, 13th edn. Churchill Livingstone Elsevier.

du Plessis, M., Zipfel, B., Brantingham, J.W., Parkin-Smith, G.F. *et al.* (2011) Manual and manipulative therapy compared to night splint for symptomatic hallux abducto valgus: An exploratory randomised clinical trial. *The Foot* 21, 2, 71–78.

Eisenhart, A.W., Gaeta, T.J. and Yens, D.P. (2003) Osteopathic manipulative treatment in the emergency department for patients with acute ankle injuries. *Journal of Osteopathic Medicine* 103, 9, 417–421.

Evans, D.W. (2002) Mechanisms and effects of spinal high-velocity, low-amplitude thrust manipulation: Previous theories. *Journal of Manipulative and Physiological Therapeutics* 25, 4, 251–262.

Evans, D.W. and Lucas, N. (2010) What is 'manipulation'? A reappraisal. *Manual Therapy* 15, 3, 286–291.

Freitas, S.M., Wieczorek, S.A., Marchetti, P.H. and Duarte, M. (2005) Age-related changes in human postural control of prolonged standing. *Gait and Posture* 22, 4, 322–330.

Gao, C.Y., Gao, J.H. and Wang, Q.F. (2015) Clinical research of rotating-traction-poking manipulation with acute lateral ankle sprains. *Zhong Guo Zhong Yi Gu Shang Ke Za Zhi* 23, 10–13.

Gevers-Montoro, C., Provencher, B., Descarreaux, M., Ortega de Mues, A. and Piché, M. (2021) Neurophysiological mechanisms of chiropractic spinal manipulation for spine pain. *European Journal of Pain* 25, 7, 1429–1448.

Gyer, G., Michael, J., Inklebarger, J. and Alam, I.I. (2021) Effects of biomechanical parameters of spinal manipulation: A critical literature review. *Journal of Integrative Medicine* 20, 1, 4–12.

Gyer, G., Michael, J., Inklebarger, J. and Tedla, J.S. (2019) Spinal manipulation therapy: Is it all about the brain? A current review of the neurophysiological effects of manipulation. *Journal of Integrative Medicine 17*, 5, 328–337.

Haavik, H. and Murphy, B. (2012) The role of spinal manipulation in addressing disordered sensorimotor integration and altered motor control. *Journal of Electromyography and Kinesiology 22*, 5, 768–776.

Harris, S.R. (1996) How should treatments be critiqued for scientific merit? *Physical Therapy 76*, 2, 175–181.

Hattam, P. and Smeatham, A. (2010) *Special Tests in Musculoskeletal Examination: An Evidence-Based Guide for Clinicians*. Churchill Livingstone Elsevier.

Hoskins, W., McHardy, A., Pollard, H., Windsham, R. and Onley, R. (2006) Chiropractic treatment of lower extremity conditions: A literature review. *Journal of Manipulative Physiological Therapeutics 29*, 8, 658–671.

Kamani, N.C., Poojari, S. and Prabu, R.G. (2021) The influence of fascial manipulation on function, ankle dorsiflexion range of motion and postural sway in individuals with chronic ankle instability. *Journal of Bodywork and Movement Therapies 27*, 216–221.

Lavery, L.A., Armstrong, D.G. and Boulton, A.J. (2002) Ankle equinus deformity and its relationship to high plantar pressure in a large population with diabetes mellitus. *Journal of the American Podiatric Medical Association 92*, 9, 479–482.

Lelic, D., Niazi, I.K., Holt, K., Jochumsen, M. *et al.* (2016) Manipulation of dysfunctional spinal joints affects sensorimotor integration in the prefrontal cortex: A brain source localization study. *Neural Plasticity 2016*, 3704964.

Lin, C.W.C., Hiller, C.E. and De Bie, R.A. (2010) Evidence-based treatment for ankle injuries: A clinical perspective. *Journal of Manual and Manipulative Therapy 18*, 1, 22–28.

López-Rodríguez, S., de-Las-Peñas, C.F., Alburquerque-Sendín, F., Rodríguez-Blanco, C. and Palomeque-del-Cerro, L. (2007) Immediate effects of manipulation of the talocrural joint on stabilometry and baropodometry in patients with ankle sprain. *Journal of Manipulative and Physiological Therapeutics 30*, 3, 186–192.

Loudon, J.K., Reiman, M.P. and Sylvain, J. (2014) The efficacy of manual joint mobilisation/manipulation in treatment of lateral ankle sprains: A systematic review. *British Journal of Sports Medicine 48*, 5, 365–370.

Machado, Á.S., Silva, C.B.P.D., Rocha, E.S.D. and Carpes, F.P. (2017) Effects of plantar foot sensitivity manipulation on postural control of young adult and elderly. *Revista Brasileira de Reumatologia 57*, 30–36.

Magee, D.J. (2014) *Orthopedic Physical Assessment*, 6th edn. Saunders.

Malanga, G.A., Andrus, S., Nadler, S.F. and McLean, J. (2003) Physical examination of the knee: A review of the original test description and scientific validity of common orthopedic tests. *Archives of Physical Medicine and Rehabilitation 84*, 592–603.

Manske, R.C. and Prohaska, D. (2008) Physical examination and imaging of the acute multiple ligament knee injury. *North American Journal of Sports Physical Therapy 3*, 4, 191–197.

Melzack, R. and Wall, P.D. (1967) Pain mechanisms: A new theory. *Survey of Anesthesiology 11*, 2, 89–90.

Menz, H.B. (1998) Manipulative therapy of the foot and ankle: Science or mesmerism? *The Foot 8*, 2, 68–74.

Mortka, K. and Lisiński, P. (2015) Hallux valgus – a case for a physiotherapist or only for a surgeon? Literature review. *Journal of Physical Therapy Science 27*, 10, 3303–3307.

Ostrowski, J.A. (2006) Accuracy of 3 diagnostic tests for anterior cruciate ligament tears. *Journal of Athletic Training 41*, 1, 120–121.

Pellow, J.E. and Brantingham, J.W. (2001) The efficacy of adjusting the ankle in the treatment of subacute and chronic grade I and grade II ankle inversion sprains. *Journal of Manipulative and Physiological Therapeutics 24*, 1, 17–24.

Pickar, J.G. (2002) Neurophysiological effects of spinal manipulation. *The Spine Journal* 2, 5, 357–371.

Polkinghorn, B.S. (1995) Posterior calcaneal subluxation: An important consideration in chiropractic treatment of plantar fasciitis (heel spur syndrome). *Chiropractic Sports Medicine* 9, 44–51.

Pollack, Y., Shashua, A. and Kalichman, L. (2018) Manual therapy for plantar heel pain. *The Foot* 34, 11–16.

Polzer, H., Polzer, S., Brumann, M., Mutschler, W. and Regauer, M. (2014) Hallux rigidus: Joint preserving alternatives to arthrodesis – a review of the literature. *World Journal of Orthopedics* 5, 1, 6–13.

Randoll, C., Gagnon-Normandin, V., Tessier, J., Bois, S. *et al.* (2017) The mechanism of back pain relief by spinal manipulation relies on decreased temporal summation of pain. *Neuroscience* 349, 220–228.

Roston, J.B. and Haines, R.W. (1947) Cracking in the metacarpo-phalangeal joint. *Journal of Anatomy* 81, 2, 165–173.

Sandoz, R. (1976) Some physical mechanisms and effects of spinal adjustments. *Annals of the Swiss Chiropracters' Association* 6, 2, 91–142.

Savva, C., Giakas, G. and Efstathiou, M. (2014) The role of the descending inhibitory pain mechanism in musculoskeletal pain following high-velocity, low-amplitude thrust manipulation: A review of the literature. *Journal of Back and Musculoskeletal Rehabilitation* 27, 4, 377–382.

Schuh, R., Hofstaetter, S.G., Adams Jr, S.B., Pichler, F., Kristen, K.H. and Trnka, H.J. (2009) Rehabilitation after hallux valgus surgery: Importance of physical therapy to restore weight bearing of the first ray during the stance phase. *Physical Therapy* 89, 9, 934–945.

Schwartz, E.N. and Su, J. (2014) Plantar fasciitis: A concise review. *The Permanente Journal* 18, 1, e105.

Schwieterman, B., Haas, D., Columber, K., Knupp, D. and Cook, C. (2013) Diagnostic accuracy of physical examination tests of the ankle/foot complex: A systematic review. *International Journal of Sports Physical Therapy* 8, 4, 416–426.

Shamus, J., Shamus, E., Gugel, R.N., Brucker, B.S. and Skaruppa, C. (2004) The effect of sesamoid mobilization, flexor hallucis strengthening, and gait training on reducing pain and restoring function in individuals with hallux limitus: A clinical trial. *Journal of Orthopaedic and Sports Physical Therapy* 34, 7, 368–376.

Shin, H.J., Kim, S.H., Jung, H.J., Cho, H.Y. and Hahm, S.C. (2020) Manipulative therapy plus ankle therapeutic exercises for adolescent baseball players with chronic ankle instability: A single-blinded randomized controlled trial. *International Journal of Environmental Research and Public Health* 17, 14, 4997.

Sibley, K.M., Beauchamp, M.K., Van Ooteghem, K., Straus, S.E. and Jaglal, S.B. (2015) Using the systems framework for postural control to analyze the components of balance evaluated in standardized balance measures: A scoping review. *Archives of Physical Medicine and Rehabilitation* 96, 1, 122–132.

Slaughter, A.J., Reynolds, K.A., Jambhekar, K., David, R.M., Hasan, S.A. and Pandey, T. (2014) Clinical orthopedic examination findings in the lower extremity: Correlation with imaging studies and diagnostic efficacy. *RadioGraphics* 34, 2, e41–e55.

Staud, R., Craggs, J.G., Robinson, M.E., Perlstein, W.M. and Price, D.D. (2007) Brain activity related to temporal summation of C-fiber evoked pain. *Pain* 129, 1–2, 130–142.

Stephenson, C. (2013) *The Complementary Therapist's Guide to Red Flags and Referrals.* Churchill Livingstone Elsevier.

Truyols-Domínguez, S., Salom-Moreno, J., Abian-Vicen, J., Cleland, J.A. and Fernández-de-Las-Peñas, C. (2013) Efficacy of thrust and nonthrust manipulation and exercise with or without the addition of myofascial therapy for the management of acute inversion ankle sprain: A randomized clinical trial. *Journal of Orthopaedic and Sports Physical Therapy* 43, 5, 300–309.

Unsworth, A., Dowson, D. and Wright, V. (1971) 'Cracking joints': A bioengineering study of cavitation in the metacarpophalangeal joint. *Annals of the Rheumatic Diseases 30*, 4, 348–358.

Vaillant, J., Vuillerme, N., Janvey, A., Louis, F. *et al.* (2008) Effect of manipulation of the feet and ankles on postural control in elderly adults. *Brain Research Bulletin 75*, 1, 18–22.

Van der Wees, P.J., Lenssen, A.F., Hendriks, E.J., Stomp, D.J., Dekker, J. and de Bie, R.A. (2006) Effectiveness of exercise therapy and manual mobilisation in acute ankle sprain and functional instability: A systematic review. *Australian Journal of Physiotherapy 52*, 1, 27–37.

Van Ochten, J.M., van Middelkoop, M., Meuffels, D. and Bierma-Zeinstra, S.M. (2014) Chronic complaints after ankle sprains: A systematic review on effectiveness of treatments. *Journal of Orthopaedic and Sports Physical Therapy 44*, 11, 862–871.

Vernon, H. and Mrozek, J. (2005) A revised definition of manipulation. *Journal of Manipulative and Physiological Therapeutics 28*, 1, 68–72.

Wang, B., Yin, X., Zhang, P., Yang, K. *et al.* (2021) Effect of traditional Chinese manipulation on ankle sprains: A systematic review and meta-analysis. *Medicine 100*, 5, e24065.

Whitman, J.M., Cleland, J.A., Mintken, P., Keirns, M. *et al.* (2009) Predicting short-term response to thrust and nonthrust manipulation and exercise in patients post inversion ankle sprain. *Journal of Orthopaedic and Sports Physical Therapy 39*, 3, 188–200.

Wise, C.H. (2015) *Orthopaedic Manual Physical Therapy: From Art to Evidence.* F.A. Davis Company.

World Health Organization (WHO) (2005) *WHO Guidelines on Basic Training and Safety in Chiropractic.* WHO, www.wfc.org/website/index.php?option=com_content&view=article&id=110&lang=en

Yelverton, C., Rama, S. and Zipfel, B. (2019) Manual therapy interventions in the treatment of plantar fasciitis: A comparison of three approaches. *Health SA 24*, 1244.

Chapter 11

Dry Needling of the Foot and Ankle

Over recent decades, dry needling has become an increasingly popular treatment technique in manual therapy practice. Physical therapy practitioners from various disciplines such as chiropractic, osteopathy and physiotherapy today utilise dry needling in the clinical management of various neuromusculoskeletal conditions, particularly myofascial pain and trigger points (TrPs) (Dommerholt, 2011). TrPs, also called myofascial trigger points (MTrPs), are hyperirritable or hypersensitive spots that are usually located in the palpable taut bands of skeletal muscle. TrPs become painful upon palpation and are associated with a local twitch response (LTR), local pain and tenderness, referred pain and tenderness, motor dysfunction, increased muscle fatigability and autonomic phenomena. TrPs are also peripheral sources of constant nociceptive input to the brain, which ultimately lead to peripheral and central sensitisation (Alvarez and Rockwell, 2002; Lavelle *et al.*, 2007; Dommerholt, 2011).

The positive effects of dry needling in the management of TrPs are increasingly documented in the literature (Dunning *et al.*, 2014). Dry needling has been shown to reduce local and referred pain, restore range of motion, improve muscle activation patterns and alter the chemical environment of active TrPs (Shah *et al.*, 2003; Hsieh *et al.*, 2007; Shah *et al.*, 2008; Fernández-Carnero *et al.*, 2010; Al-Boloushi *et al.*, 2020; Geist *et al.*, 2021). There is also evidence that dry needling can normalise some aspects of peripheral and central sensitisation (Affaitati *et al.*, 2011; Dommerholt, 2011; Fernández-de-Las-Peñas and Nijs, 2019). These findings provide some evidence in support of the long-held notion that it may be an instrumental intervention in treating TrPs by neutralising the persistent nociceptive source.

Dry needling has also been suggested to be a potential intervention in the treatment of several foot and ankle pathologies, particularly ankle sprains, chronic ankle instability and plantar heel pain or plantar fasciitis (Cotchett *et al.*, 2010; Cotchett *et al.*, 2011; López-González *et al.*, 2021). There is an emerging theory that TrPs are exacerbated in the ankle and foot musculature following repetitive strain activities, and that this can affect motor control strategies and neuromuscular adaptation of the corresponding muscles (Mullins *et al.*, 2021b). Evidence is still limited, but previous investigations have shown abnormalities of the fibularis longus and brevis muscles in patients with ankle instability, including reduced reaction time, weakened postural control, decreased corticomotor excitability and the presence of TrPs (Pietrosimone and Gribble, 2012; Méndez-Rebolledo *et al.*, 2015; Salom-Moreno *et al.*, 2015). Therefore, if TrPs are effectively neutralised in the affected musculature, it is possible to minimise these motor disturbances by blocking overload that may spread over the surrounding structures.

Ongoing research is currently investigating outcomes of dry needling in combination with the standard of care for ankle and foot conditions. Although it is too early to reach a conclusion, the available evidence indicates that dry needling combined with a conventional rehabilitation approach can yield superior outcomes in pain relief and functional improvement (Salom-Moreno *et al.*, 2015; Rossi *et al.*, 2017; Mullins *et al.*, 2021a). This chapter therefore provides a general overview of dry needling: what it is, how it works and its clinical relevance in the treatment of ankle and foot conditions.

What is dry needling?

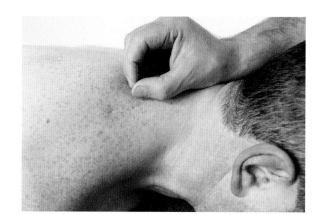

Dry needling is an intervention that involves the insertion of thin filiform needles – similar to acupuncture practice – into TrP or non-TrP sites without any injectate. The intervention primarily aims to reduce pain and dysfunction in patients with neuromuscular pain syndromes. It can be performed at both deep and superficial tissue levels. The deep needling technique targets primarily dysfunctional motor end plates, while the superficial technique is aimed mostly at peripheral sensory afferents (Dommerholt, 2011; Fernández-de-Las-Peñas and Nijs, 2019).

- **The American Physical Therapy Association (APTA) definition:** Dry needling is a skilled intervention that utilises thin filiform needles for skin penetration and, in turn, stimulation of underlying MTrPs, muscular and connective tissues to treat various neuromusculoskeletal disorders (APTA, 2013).

- **The Australian Society of Acupuncture Physiotherapists (ASAP) definition:** Dry needling is the short-term insertion of needles into dysfunctional tissues to reduce pain and restore function. The needling may be targeted at MTrPs, periosteum and connective tissues (ASAP, 2014).

There are various types of dry needling. One of the popular types is the insertion of needles targeting only the TrPs, which is more commonly referred to as TrP dry needling. Another popular form is the combination of dry needling with electrical current, which is commonly known as percutaneous electrolysis or electric dry needling (Dommerholt and Fernández-de-las-Peñas, 2018; Dunning *et al.*, 2018).

Controversy

In recent years, there has been a concerted effort among various physical therapy professional organisations to narrow the definition of dry needling to a TrP or 'intramuscular' procedure. Some have even equated the definition with the term TrP dry needling or intramuscular manual therapy (IMT). However, although the needling of TrPs within muscle bellies is critically important to induce therapeutic benefits, it is just an individual aspect of dry needling. In fact, the needling of non-TrP sites is supported by a large body of literature, including randomised controlled trials and systematic reviews. Thus, the term TrP dry needling or IMT cannot be used synonymously with the term dry needling, as each represents an individual approach that falls under the umbrella of dry needling (Dunning *et al.*, 2014).

How dry needling works

The underlying mechanisms through which dry needling works are still largely unknown. The scientific community has so far proposed both biomechanical and neurophysiological mechanisms for the observed therapeutic effects of dry needling. However, these theorised mechanisms are primarily based on the motor and neural components of the TrPs.

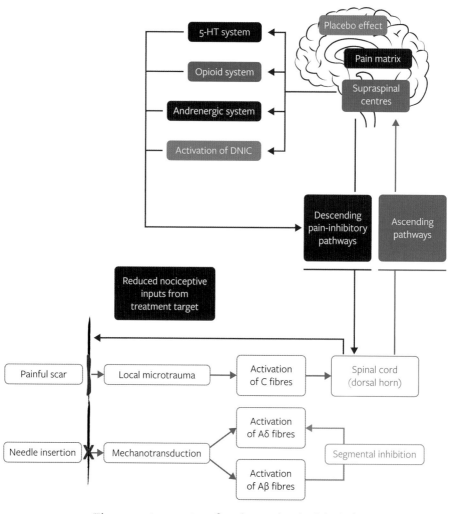

Figure 11.1 Acupuncture flowchart – the physiological mechanisms of acupuncture-induced analgesia

Blue arrows = activation; red arrows = inhibition.

5-HT = 5-hydroxtryptamine; DNIC = diffuse noxious inhibitory control.

Biomechanical mechanisms

The proposed biomechanical mechanisms of dry needling are largely based on the radiculopathy model by Gunn (1997). This model is founded upon Cannon and Rosenblueth's (1949) Law of Denervation, which states that the free flow of nerve impulses is essential for a regulatory or trophic effect; however, this free flow depends primarily on the functional integrity of innervated structures. Based on this law, Gunn states that the pathological neural tissue hypersensitises all innervated structures as a result of the disrupted flow of nerve impulses, and eventually leads to the development of TrPs. Gunn (2003) proposes that accurate and repeated needling of muscles may restore this flow of nerve impulses through the release of nerve root entrapment and thereby muscle contracture.

Up to now, no conclusive evidence has been found in support of the Gunn model. However, dry needling has been shown to upset the dysfunctional motor end plates and mitigate end plate noise (i.e. spontaneous electrical activity), which are often associated with TrPs (Fernández-de-Las-Peñas and Nijs, 2019). This has been confirmed by several studies, which showed a reduction in frequency and amplitude of end plate noise and spike following the application of dry needling (Chou *et al.*, 2009; Abbaszadeh-Amirdehi *et al.*, 2017; Liu *et al.*, 2017). In short, dry needling has an effect on dysfunctional motor end plates. Dry needling is also suggested to restore the extremely shortened sarcomeres to their resting length. Dommerholt (2004) hypothesised that accurate needling could induce a local stretching of the shortened skeletal muscles, which may release the entangled myosin filaments at the Z-band and, in turn, reduce the contracture of the sarcomere by inhibiting the overlapping of actin and myosin filaments. Dry needling has been shown to restore the local circulation of blood and oxygen in the pathological musculature, which provides some support for the lessening of sarcomere contracture (Cagnie *et al.*, 2012).

Furthermore, the observed spontaneous electrical activity following dry needling has been reported to be associated with the presence of LTRs (Hong, 1994; Kuan *et al.*, 2007; Hsieh *et al.*, 2011). An LTR is an involuntary spinal reflex that causes a brisk contraction of the skeletal muscle fibres in a taut band. The central nervous system modulates LTRs. The LTR is a well-known clinical feature of active TrPs (Bron and Dommerholt, 2012). LTRs are usually elicited during the application of deep dry needling and have been claimed to signify the effectiveness of the applied needling intervention (Perreault *et al.*, 2017). The elicitation of LTRs has been shown to inactivate TrPs, mitigate abnormal motor end plate noise, reduce the concentration of various nociceptors and biochemicals, normalise the chemical milieu surrounding a TrP and relax the taut band (Fernández-Carnero *et al.*, 2010; Hakim *et al.*, 2019; Al-Boloushi *et al.*, 2020; Geist *et al.*, 2021). In addition, Shah *et al.* (2003) showed that the elicitation of LTRs with dry needling immediately reduced heightened levels of numerous chemicals related to the immune system, including substance P (SP), calcitonin gene-related peptide (CGRP) and bradykinin, to name a few. From a mechanical viewpoint, Chu and Schwartz (2002) theorised that when a needle is speedily inserted into a trigger point, the elicited LTRs cause a large afferent nerve fibre proprioceptive input into the spinal cord, which could have a central effect on the pain gate in the spinal cord. This may, in turn, block the intra-dorsal horn passage, which ascends noxious signals produced by nociceptors at TrPs.

Taken together, it is apparent from the available evidence that dry needling has several mechanical effects, which consequently may trigger a series of neurophysiological mechanisms.

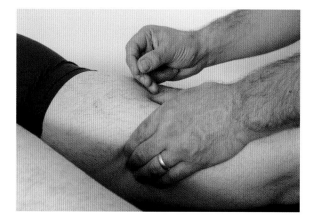

Neurophysiological mechanisms

From a neurophysiological standpoint, dry needling is thought to inhibit both peripheral and central sensitisation through a number of mechanisms, including removal of peripheral nociceptive sources (i.e. by neutralising TrPs), modulation of dorsal-horn-mediated neural activity, and activation of descending pain-inhibitory pathways (Fernández-de-Las-Peñas and Nijs, 2019). Although evidence is still limited, there is some evidence that peripheral stimulation of skin and muscles by dry needling elicits different neural responses, which are thought to induce a cascade of pain-modulatory mechanisms, mediated by the nervous system.

The first proposed mechanism is the inhibition of peripheral nociception. TrPs are well-recognised sources of constant peripheral nociceptive inputs to the CNS. As discussed above, deep dry needling inactivates TrPs by eliciting LTRs, which have been shown to alter the biochemical environment and neurotransmitter concentrations surrounding TrPs. In fact, studies by Shah *et al.* (2003, 2008) and Hsieh *et al.* (2012) reported an immediate reduction in the peripheral concentrations of different neurotransmitters (e.g. SP, CGRP, bradykinin) and an increase in β-endorphin and TNF-α levels after needle insertion.

The stimulation of the dorsal horn by dry needling is thought to activate mechanoreceptors coupled to sensory afferents, including A-beta, A-delta and unmyelinated C fibres. These nerve fibres have long been thought to mediate the gate control mechanism of pain and inhibit the nociceptive pathway at the dorsal horn by activating the descending pain-inhibitory systems (Staud and Price, 2006). In support of this theory, Cagnie *et al.* (2013) in their review suggested that rapid dry needling could activate both the large A-beta fibres and A-delta fibres, which could direct afferent impulses through the dorsolateral tracts of the spinal cord to the CNS. From the evidence standpoint, several studies have so far supported the dorsal-horn-mediated mechanism, which reported bidirectional remote effects of dry needling during unilateral needle insertion (Audette *et al.*, 2004; Srbely *et al.*, 2010; Tsai *et al.*, 2010; Hsieh *et al.*, 2014). In fact, experimenting on rabbit skeletal muscle, Hsieh *et al.* (2011) suggested that these remote effects of dry needling primarily utilise an uninterrupted afferent pathway to the spinal cord from the needle insertion site, while normal neurons in the dorsal horn function at those innervated levels of the related muscle.

Finally, the stimulation of dorsal horn neuronal activity through needling therapies has long been thought to activate many brainstem areas associated with pain-inhibitory mechanisms. It has been hypothesised that on their way to the CNS, these nerve impulses may project to the periaqueductal grey (PAG) area and neurons in the rostroventral medulla (RVM). From there, they may lead to the activation of descending pain-inhibitory pathways. This loop may involve the release of endogenous opioid peptides (enkephalins and β-endorphins), monoamines (serotonin and noradrenaline) and GABA (γ-aminobutyric acid) and glycine (Cao, 2002; Leung, 2012; Lundeberg, 2013). Evidence from the current literature also supports these proposed mechanisms. In fact, studies have shown that needling therapies could modulate relevant brain areas involved in the limbic–paralimbic–neocortical network and sensorimotor processing, including the hypothalamus, insula, medial prefrontal cortex, anterior and posterior cingular cortex, and amygdala, to name a few (Dommerholt, 2011; Chou *et al.*, 2012; Chae *et al.*, 2013; Fernández-de-Las-Peñas and Nijs, 2019). In addition, Niddam *et al.* (2007) suggested that the combination of dry needling and electric current might activate interneurons of the enkephalinergic inhibitory dorsal horn via the PAG.

Clinical application of dry needling in foot and ankle conditions

Ankle sprains and instability

Lateral ankle sprains are common injuries that occur more frequently in active people, particularly those who involve themselves in sporting and recreational activities. These sprains may lead to chronic ankle instability in about 40% of cases (Chan *et al.*, 2011). As discussed above, several studies have previously reported muscle abnormalities in patients with ankle instability. In fact, both fibularis longus and fibularis brevis muscles are known to be affected by ankle instability (Pietrosimone and Gribble, 2012; Méndez-Rebolledo *et al.*, 2015). Hence, dry needling can be a suitable treatment for ankle sprains and instability, as it can neutralise TrPs in these muscles.

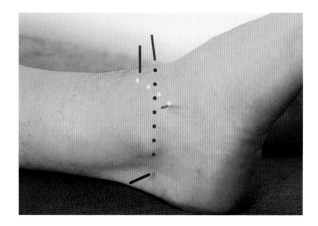

To date, evidence to support this claim is still limited. However, in a randomised controlled trial (RCT) on patients with chronic ankle instability, Salom-Moreno *et al.* (2015) found that dry needling of the fibularis muscle in combination with proprioceptive training was more effective than proprioceptive training alone for pain alleviation and functional improvement. Recently, López-González *et al.* (2021) conducted a single-blinded RCT to evaluate the effects of dry needling applied on latent TrPs in peroneus longus and tibialis anterior muscles of ankle instability patients. The authors noted enhanced neuromuscular control and improved static postural control following dry needling. Another recent study by Mullins *et al.* (2021a) also reported similar improvements in postural control outcomes in individuals with chronic ankle instability immediately following dry needling.

Plantar fasciitis

Plantar fasciitis is a degenerative disease of the plantar fascia, which causes stabbing pain in the heel and bottom of the foot. As the plantar arch has ligamentous and muscular attachments with other bony structures of the foot and ankle, the presence of TrPs is obvious, which may play an important role in pain facilitatory mechanisms (Bron and Dommerholt, 2012). Hence, dry needling can be a plausible treatment option to address plantar heel pain. A number of studies to date have evaluated the efficacy of dry needling in the management of plantar fasciitis, which predominantly reported an improvement in plantar heel pain with long-lasting effects (Cotchett *et al.*, 2010, 2011, 2014; Eftekharsadat *et al.*, 2016; Al-Boloushi *et al.*, 2020). Although these studies can be subjected to many methodological limitations, a recent meta-analysis has also confirmed the effectiveness of dry needling in reducing heel pain resulting from plantar fasciitis (He and Ma, 2017). However, more high-quality RCTs are needed to fully establish dry needling as a conventional treatment option for plantar fasciitis.

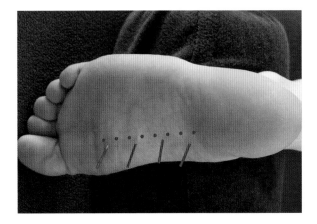

Table 11.1 Scientific evidence supporting dry needling for
the treatment of various foot and ankle conditions

Condition	Authors	Design	Clinical findings
Lateral ankle sprain	Rossi *et al.* (2017)	RCT	Patients who received dry needling of both L5 multifidi and fibularis muscles showed no improvement in strength, unilateral balance and unilateral hop test performance when compared to those who received dry needling of fibularis muscles alone. However, it appeared that fibularis muscle dry needling might temporarily improve strength and unilateral balance in patients with ankle sprains.
Chronic ankle instability	Salom-Moreno *et al.* (2015)	RCT	Dry needling of the fibularis muscle in combination with proprioceptive training was more effective than proprioceptive training alone for pain alleviation and functional improvement.
	López-González *et al.* (2021)	RCT	Dry needling applied on latent TrPs in peroneus longus and tibialis anterior muscles resulted in enhanced neuromuscular control in patients with ankle instability.
Postural control	Mullins *et al.* (2021a)	RCT	Dry needling of the fibularis longus muscle improved static and postural control in both healthy subjects and chronic ankle instability patients.
	Méndez-Rebolledo *et al.* (2015)	Case-control study	Dry needling of the fibularis and tibialis anterior muscles resulted in reduced postural control and longer reaction time in basketball players with functional ankle instability.
	López-González *et al.* (2021)	RCT	Dry needling applied on latent TrPs in peroneus longus and tibialis anterior muscles resulted in improvement in static postural control in patients with ankle instability.
Plantar fasciitis	Cotchett *et al.* (2010)	SR	Limited evidence was found in support of the effectiveness of TrP dry needling for plantar heel pain.
	Al-Boloushi *et al.* (2020)	RCT	Both dry needling and percutaneous needle electrolysis were found to be effective for the management of plantar heel pain, with long-lasting effects (52 weeks). However, the long-term outcome of percutaneous needle electrolysis was better than dry needling in terms of quality-of-life improvement.
	He and Ma (2017)	MA	Dry needling of TrPs was found to be effective in reducing heel pain due to plantar fasciitis. However, the need for more high-quality RCTs was suggested.

| Hallux valgus | Kharazmi et al. (2020) | RCT | Dry needling of TrPs demonstrated a significant decrease in hallux valgus angle in symptomatic patients. However, no statistically significant difference was reported in pain scale and foot function index between the sham intervention and dry needling. The authors recommended dry needling for improving the alignment of first ray. |
| | Ying et al. (2021) | SR & MA | Dry needling combined with other conservative treatments was identified as the best possible choice for reducing intermetatarsal and first metatarsophalangeal angles. However, more high-quality research was recommended. |

MA = meta-analysis; RCT = randomised controlled trial; SR = systematic review.

Contraindications

Absolute contraindications

Dry needling is absolutely contraindicated in several circumstances (APTA, 2013; ASAP, 2014). These include:

- Patients having a needle aversion or needle phobia.
- Patients unwilling to be treated with dry needling.
- Patients with local or systemic infections.
- Patients unable to give consent due to significant cognitive impairment, communication difficulty or age-related factors.
- Patients allergic to nickel or chromium needles. In such cases, silver- or gold-plated needles should be used.
- Presence of local lymphoedema over an area or limb.
- Patients presenting with an acute medical condition.
- Patients unsuitable for any other valid reason.

Relative contraindications

- Severe hyperalgesia or allodynia.
- Compromised immune system.

- Presence of local skin lesions on the application site.

- Abnormal bleeding tendency.

- First trimester of pregnancy.

- Presence of vascular disease.

- Diabetes.

- Epilepsy.

Therapists should be aware that the foot and ankle is a sensitive area for the use of dry needling. The skin should be cleaned prior to needling techniques, with no oils or creams on the skin.

Dry needling techniques for the foot and ankle

Gastrocnemius and soleus

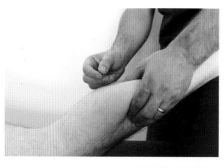

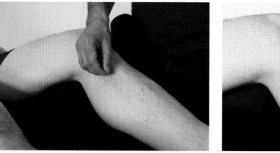

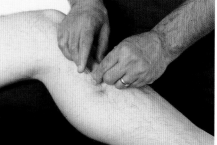

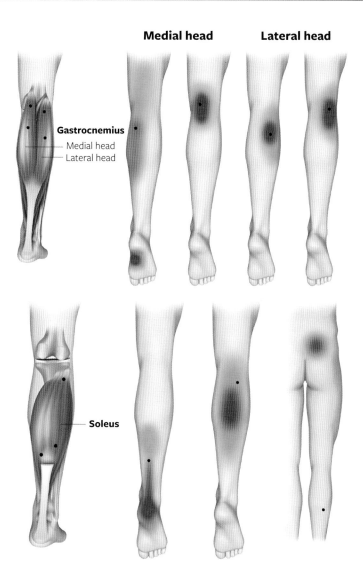

Palpation: The gastrocnemius and soleus muscles are located in the calf region and are known as the tricep surae muscles. The muscles work together as plantar flexors, which bend the foot back at the ankle joint. This also causes the leg to flex at the knee and results in propulsion and stabilisation. The gastrocnemius is the largest calf muscle and is positioned over the soleus muscle.

The gastrocnemius originates from the knee and runs to the ankle joint. It has two parallel muscle bellies that merge together mid-calf. The soleus has multiple origin points, with fibres merging into a large tendon and inserting into the heel bone. Palpate the entire length of the calf. Extend the knee in prone position and resist. Palpate the medial and lateral heads and the attachment on the heel.

Pain referral pattern: The gastrocnemius and soleus muscles have an extended pain referral pattern for the whole of the calf region, including the outside calf. Pain concentrates in the instep of the foot and can also extend upwards to the back of the thigh. Secondary pain is referred to the back of the knee.

Needling technique: With the patient in a prone or side-lying position, palpate the gastrocnemius muscle and locate specific points of pain, needling at a perpendicular angle into the centre bulk of the muscle. With the soleus, palpate and locate the target area, and insert the needle either in the lateral or the medial side of the calf and needle towards the soleus.

Clinical implications: There are several nerves which run through the lower extremity and these should be avoided. If the patient feels an electrical referral, then the needles should be removed and replaced slightly away from the painful spot.

Popliteus

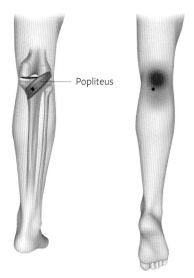

Popliteus

Palpation: The popliteus muscle originates from three points – the lateral femoral condyle, fibula and posterior horn of the lateral meniscus. The muscle rises from the proximal tibia and inserts into the posterior surface of the tibia, above the soleus. The thin and flat triangular popliteus muscle wraps around the lower section of the femur and provides flexion of the knee joint and lateral rotation of the femur. The muscle is most accessible at the lower medial end and upper lateral end of the muscle belly. With the patient in the prone position, palpate directly between the semitendinosus tendon and medial head of the gastrocnemius muscle. Flex the knee and the foot at the ankle to slacken the muscles. The soleus muscle can be laterally displaced to partially uncover the popliteus.

> **Pain referral pattern:** Popliteus primary pain referral is localised in the leg, ankle and foot, and refers posterior knee pain.

> **Needling technique:** With the patient in either a prone or side-lying position, locate the muscle behind the posterior aspect of the knee. Use an inferior needling technique to needle the muscle laterally, avoiding deep perpendicular needling of the posterior knee.

> **Clinical implications:** The therapist must be aware of the neurovascular bundle which sits just behind the popliteus muscle. Using an inferior technique to needle the muscle laterally avoids contacting this delicate structure. If the patient does feel a strong referral from the nerve, then remove and replace the needle.

Plantaris

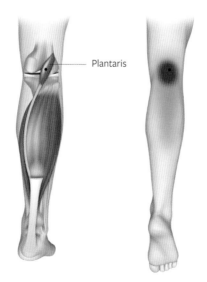

Plantaris

Palpation: The small plantaris muscle is located in the posterior aspect of the leg and forms part of the posterosuperficial compartment of the calf. Along with the gastrocnemius and soleus, the thin muscle belly and long thin tendon makes up the triceps surae muscle.

The plantaris originates from the lateral supracondylar line of the femur and from the oblique popliteal ligament located in the posterior aspect of the knee. Palpation of the muscle is possible in the popliteal fossa and the medial aspect of the common tendon. With the patient in prone position, flex the leg and cover the heel with the distal hand. Use the forearm to create resistance for the foot and knee flexion. Palpate the muscle in the popliteal fossa and Achilles tendon.

> **Pain referral pattern:** The plantaris primarily refers pain in the posterior aspect and plantar surface of the heel. This can include the distal end of the Achilles tendon and the sacroiliac joints on the same side of the body. Pain is referred to the posterior of the knee and into the calf region.

> **Needling technique:** Locate the upper lateral head of the gastrocnemius muscle and locate the plantaris muscle. The therapist can needle into the muscle either in a perpendicular or lateral direction.

> **Clinical implications:** Exercise caution around the tibial and peroneal nerves. If the patient feels a strong referral, then the needle should be removed and replaced nearby.

Tibialis anterior and posterior

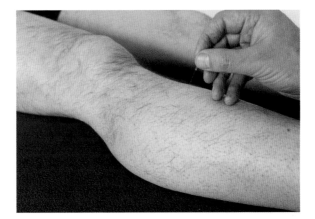

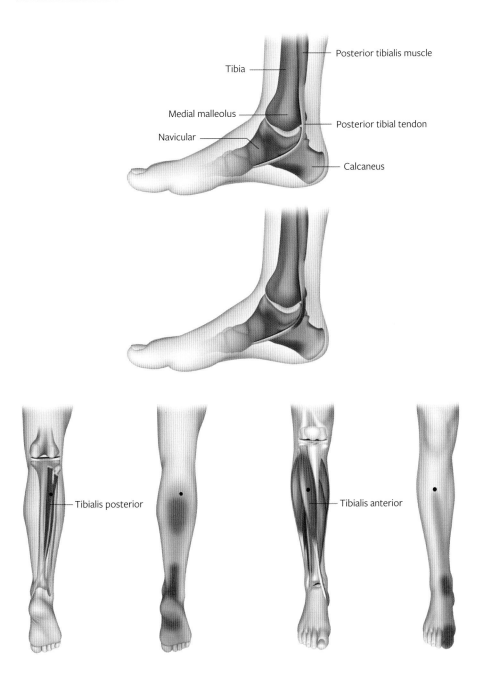

Palpation: The tibialis anterior is located in the front of the leg. The large superficial muscle originates close to the lateral tibial condyle and inserts on the foot. Together with the peroneus longus, which inserts at the base of the foot, the tibialis anterior forms a stirrup that loops around the midfoot. The muscles control movement of the foot.

The tibialis anterior adjusts its function according to the position of the foot and also supports the medial arch. To palpate, stand at the feet and use the thumb to locate the lateral edge of the tibial shaft. Laterally slide on to the muscle belly and continue to palpate towards the front of the ankle and arch. Resist for ankle dorsiflexion and inversion.

Pain referral pattern: As a great deal of stress is put on the front of the tibialis anterior, pain is referred to the shin, ankle or foot. The pain starts gradually and can worsen over time due to aggravating activity. The tibialis interior tendon is a secondary referral site.

Needling technique: Once identified, with the patient either supine or side-lying, locate the bulk of the tibialis anterior or needle directly into any tender spots identified in a perpendicular manner. Angle the needle in a slightly medial direction towards the tibia to avoid the underlying neurovascular bundle.

Clinical implications: Deep to the tibialis anterior lies the peroneal nerve and the tibial artery and vein; by needling at a medial angle, the therapist will limit/avoid this structure.

Peroneals

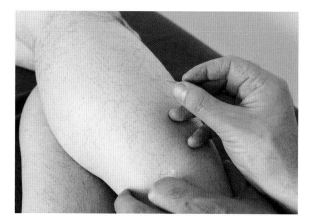

Peroneus longus   **Peroneus brevis**   **Peroneus tertius**

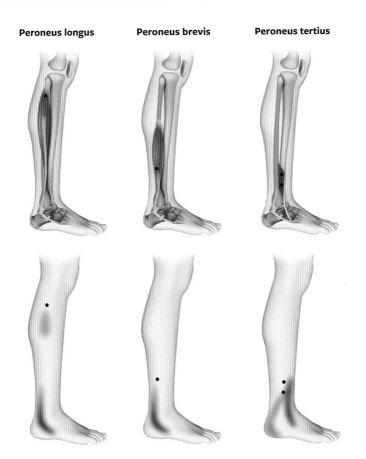

Palpation: The peroneal muscle group is made up of two muscles – peroneus longus and peroneus brevis – and is located within the peroneal compartment, in the lower leg region. The muscles can be easily seen when the foot is lowered, as they form the surface of the lateral lower leg. The muscle tendons run towards the foot behind the lateral malleolus and ventrally along the edge of the foot. Peroneus longus and peroneus brevis are responsible for moving the upper and lower ankle joints. Palpate the hollow behind the malleolus and the tendons that pass under and over the peroneal tubercle. The brevis can be palpated to its insertion.

Pain referral pattern: The primary peroneal pain refers over the lateral malleolus of the ankle and over the lateral aspect of the foot and lateral heel region. The outside edge of the shin is a secondary referral site.

Needling technique: Locate the muscle belly and angle the needle towards the fibular with the needle being inserted at a perpendicular angle towards the skin.

Clinical implications: A caution is the location of the common peroneal nerve which sits underneath the muscle; the more superficial peroneus nerve also lies within the area. The therapist should avoid direct contact with the nerve; if the patient indicates a strong electrical referral, then the needle should be removed and replaced nearby.

Achilles tendon

A simple protocol, which can be effective, is to use a four-needle cross-pattern technique. Two needles are inserted near the insertion of the Achilles and the other pair are inserted superiorly to this, still within the Achilles tendon. These can be left in situ with no stimulation to help to improve pain reduction and vascularisation. Electro acupuncture (EA) can also be used where current can be applied to cross the Achilles.

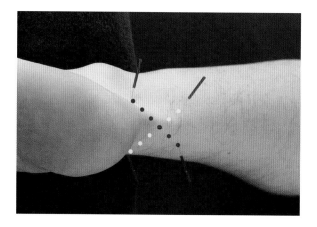

Inversion sprain

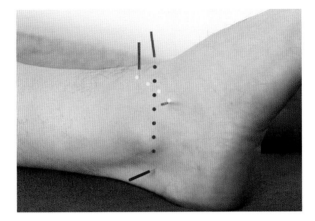

The following points are used:

- **Gallbladder 40** (anterior and inferior to the external malleolus, in the depression on the lateral side of the tendon of extensor digitorum longus) is paired with non-acupuncture points anterior to the lateral malleolus between the tibialis anterior tendon, shown with the red dotted line.

- **Stomach 41** (in the depression at the midpoint of the transverse crease of the ankle between the tendons m. extensor hallucis longus and digitorum longus) is paired with **Bladder 60** (midway between the high point of the outer ankle bone and the Achilles tendon), shown with the yellow dotted line.

This creates a cross-pattern technique across the common ligaments often involved in inversion sprains.

Herringbone technique

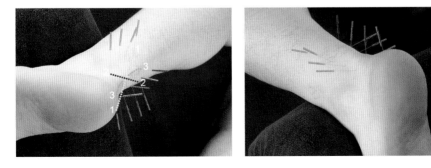

For mid-portion Achilles tendinopathy, the herringbone technique is recommended. This method has recently been adapted by acupuncturists and is beginning to be referred to as the herringbone technique because of its appearance. The configuration is achieved by inserting needles vertically, medially and laterally (i.e. parallel) to the tendon. The herringbone technique is mainly used in the Achilles tendon because of its accessibility, and it is taught on acupuncture courses. The standard method of this technique often involves the insertion of 9–12 needles vertically, medially and laterally, at equal distances from each other. The needles penetrate the tendon to a depth of around 4 mm. Measurements only serve as a guide as there are differences from patient to patient. Additional needling may be beneficial to the soleus and gastrocnemius (posterior chain), points such as Bladder 58, 57, 56, 55 and segmental points, inner/outer Bladder points and huatuojiaji points. EA can be applied in a cross pattern and along the vertical portion of the tendon using an additional pair.

For insertional tendinopathy, the herringbone technique can be used with the addition of periosteal pecking into the calcaneal insertion.

Percutaneous tenotomy and acupuncture scraping technique

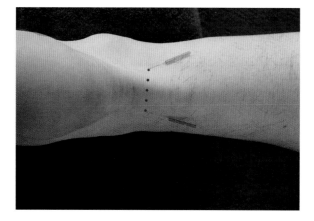

A simple technique to replicate this is to use a wide gauge needle (.30) and to lift and thrust the needle along the Achilles tendon both medially and laterally. The needle is inserted at the myotendinous junction where the gastrocnemius blends into the Achilles tendon. After lifting and thrusting, the needles can be left in place and EA can be applied, with the aim to restart the healing process.

Heel pain and plantar fasciitis

For heel pain, a four-needle cross-pattern technique can be used. Each needle is inserted into the tissue of the heel, two on the lateral side of the heel and two on the medial side of the heel. Needle insertion can be painful, so press hard on the guide tube and insert the needle quickly, causing minimal discomfort. EA can then be applied to run diagonally across the heel.

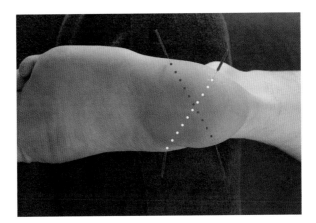

For pain in the plantar fascia, needle into the band itself, usually on the medial side. Two or four needles can be used, depending on patient tolerance. EA can be applied to the superior and inferior needles so that the current runs through the band of tissue.

If shortened calf muscles are part of the clinical picture, then needling these muscles can be included in the treatment plan (e.g. Bladder 55/56/57/58).

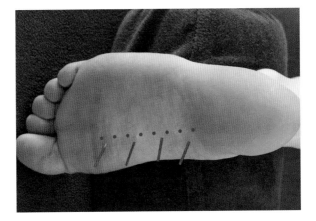

Tibialis posterior syndrome

Typically tibialis posterior tendinopathy is classified into four stages:

- **Stage 1:** Medial malleolus pain, swelling along the tendon. The patient is able to stand on tiptoe on one leg and treatment is conservative, usually with insoles and manual therapy. In the later stages, the patient will have developed an acquired flatfoot deformity.

- **Stage 2:** The patient will have increased pain and swelling compared with stage 1, increased flattening of the foot. The patient will have decreased power in the tendon. Tendon reconstruction may be necessary if conservative treatment fails.

- **Stage 3:** A degree of deformity at the subtalar joint is found on X-ray. Treated with the use of orthoses. A fusion of the hindfoot may be necessary.

- **Stage 4:** Accompanying ankle deformity. Surgery to the ankle may also be necessary.

Acupuncture technique

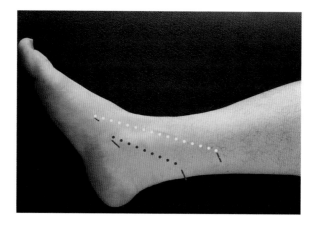

Acupuncture may be of use in tendon regeneration and pain reduction primarily in stages 1 and 2, alongside conservative management, whereas in stages 3 and 4 its use is mainly for pain management. Use the suggested points to create a cross pattern and to increase blood flow to the tendon:

- Kidney 2 to Kidney 7

- Spleen 4 to Spleen 6.

EA can be applied to stimulate a greater area across the tendon from Kidney 2 to Kidney 7 and from Spleen 4 to Spleen 6. Check for trigger points in the peroneals and lateral leg muscles.

References

Abbaszadeh-Amirdehi, M., Ansari, N.N., Naghdi, S., Olyaei, G. and Nourbakhsh, M.R. (2017) Therapeutic effects of dry needling in patients with upper trapezius myofascial trigger points. *Acupuncture in Medicine* 35, 2, 85–92.

Affaitati, G., Costantini, R., Fabrizio, A., Lapenna, D., Tafuri, E. and Giamberardino, M.A. (2011) Effects of treatment of peripheral pain generators in fibromyalgia patients. *European Journal of Pain* 15, 1, 61–69.

Al-Boloushi, Z., Gómez-Trullén, E.M., Arian, M., Fernández, D., Herrero, P. and Bellosta-López, P. (2020) Comparing two dry needling interventions for plantar heel pain: A randomised controlled trial. *BMJ Open* 10, 8, e038033.

Alvarez, D.J. and Rockwell, P.G. (2002) Trigger points: Diagnosis and management. *American Family Physician* 65, 4, 653.

APTA (2013) *Description of Dry Needling in Clinical Practice: An Educational Resource Paper.* APTA Public Policy, Practice, and Professional Affairs Unit.

ASAP (2014) *Guidelines for Safe Acupuncture and Dry Needling Practice.* Australian Society of Acupuncture Physiotherapists (ASAP).

Audette, J.F., Wang, F. and Smith, H. (2004) Bilateral activation of motor unit potentials with unilateral needle stimulation of active myofascial trigger points. *American Journal of Physical Medicine and Rehabilitation* 83, 5, 368–374.

Bron, C. and Dommerholt, J.D. (2012) Etiology of myofascial trigger points. *Current Pain and Headache Reports* 16, 5, 439–444.

Cagnie, B., Barbe, T., De Ridder, E., Van Oosterwijck, J., Cools, A. and Danneels, L. (2012) The influence of dry needling of the trapezius muscle on muscle blood flow and oxygenation. *Journal of Manipulative and Physiological Therapeutics* 35, 9, 685–691.

Cagnie, B., Dewitte, V., Barbe, T., Timmermans, F., Delrue, N. and Meeus, M. (2013) Physiologic effects of dry needling. *Current Pain and Headache Reports* 17, 8, 1–8.

Cannon, W.B. and Rosenblueth, A. (1949) *The Supersensitivity of Denervated Structures: A Law of Denervation.* Macmillan Company.

Cao, X. (2002) Scientific bases of acupuncture analgesia. *Acupuncture and Electrotherapy Research* 27, 1–14.

Chae, Y., Chang, D.S., Lee, S.H., Jung, W.M. *et al.* (2013) Inserting needles into the body: A meta-analysis of brain activity associated with acupuncture needle stimulation. *The Journal of Pain* 14, 3, 215–222.

Chan, K.W., Ding, B.C. and Mroczek, K.J. (2011) Acute and chronic lateral ankle instability in the athlete. *Bulletin of the NYU Hospital for Joint Diseases* 69, 1, 17–26.

Chou, L.W., Hsieh, Y.L., Kao, M.J. and Hong, C.Z. (2009) Remote influences of acupuncture on the pain intensity and the amplitude changes of endplate noise in the myofascial trigger point of the upper trapezius muscle. *Archives of Physical Medicine and Rehabilitation* 90, 6, 905–912.

Chou, L.W., Kao, M.J. and Lin, J.G. (2012) Probable mechanisms of needling therapies for myofascial pain control. *Evidence-Based Complementary and Alternative Medicine* 2012, 705327.

Chu, J. and Schwartz, I. (2002) The muscle twitch in myofascial pain relief: Effects of acupuncture and other needling methods. *Electromyography and Clinical Neurophysiology 42*, 5, 307–311.

Cotchett, M.P., Landorf, K.B. and Munteanu, S.E. (2010) Effectiveness of dry needling and injections of myofascial trigger points associated with plantar heel pain: A systematic review. *Journal of Foot and Ankle Research 3*, 1, 1–9.

Cotchett, M.P., Landorf, K.B., Munteanu, S.E. and Raspovic, A. (2011) Effectiveness of trigger point dry needling for plantar heel pain: Study protocol for a randomised controlled trial. *Journal of Foot and Ankle Research 4*, 1, 1–10.

Cotchett, M.P., Munteanu, S.E. and Landorf, K.B. (2014) Effectiveness of trigger point dry needling for plantar heel pain: A randomized controlled trial. *Physical Therapy 94*, 8, 1083–1094.

Dommerholt, J. (2004) Dry needling in orthopedic physical therapy practice. *Orthopaedic Physical Therapy Practice 16*, 3, 15–20.

Dommerholt, J. (2011) Dry needling – peripheral and central considerations. *Journal of Manual and Manipulative Therapy 19*, 4, 223–227.

Dommerholt, J. and Fernández-de-las-Peñas, C. (2018) *Trigger Point Dry Needling E-Book: An Evidence and Clinical-Based Approach.* Elsevier Health Sciences.

Dunning, J., Butts, R., Henry, N., Mourad, F. *et al.* (2018) Electrical dry needling as an adjunct to exercise, manual therapy and ultrasound for plantar fasciitis: A multi-center randomized clinical trial. *PLOS ONE 13*, 10, e0205405.

Dunning, J., Butts, R., Mourad, F., Young, I., Flannagan, S. and Perreault, T. (2014) Dry needling: A literature review with implications for clinical practice guidelines. *Physical Therapy Reviews 19*, 4, 252–265.

Eftekharsadat, B., Babaei-Ghazani, A. and Zeinolabedinzadeh, V. (2016) Dry needling in patients with chronic heel pain due to plantar fasciitis: A single-blinded randomized clinical trial. *Medical Journal of the Islamic Republic of Iran 30*, 401.

Fernández-Carnero, J., La Touche, R., Ortega-Santiago, R., Galan-del-Rio, F. *et al.* (2010) Short-term effects of dry needling of active myofascial trigger points in the masseter muscle in patients with temporomandibular disorders. *Journal of Orofacial Pain 24*, 1, 106–112.

Fernández-de-Las-Peñas, C. and Nijs, J. (2019) Trigger point dry needling for the treatment of myofascial pain syndrome: Current perspectives within a pain neuroscience paradigm. *Journal of Pain Research 12*, 1899–1911.

Geist, K.T., Frierson, E.M., Goudiss, H.L., Kitchen, H. *et al.* (2021) Short-term effects of dry needling at a spinal and peripheral site on functional outcome measures, strength, and proprioception among individuals with a lateral ankle sprain. *Journal of Bodywork and Movement Therapies 26*, 158–166.

Gunn, C.C. (1997) Radiculopathic pain: Diagnosis and treatment of segmental irritation or sensitization. *Journal of Musculoskeletal Pain 5*, 4, 119–134.

Gunn, C.C. (2003) *Intramuscular Stimulation (IMS) – The Technique.* www.istop.org/papers/imspaper.pdf

Hakim, I.K., Takamjani, I.E., Sarrafzadeh, J., Ezzati, K. and Bagheri, R. (2019) The effect of dry needling on the active trigger point of upper trapezius muscle: Eliciting local twitch response on long-term clinical outcomes. *Journal of Back and Musculoskeletal Rehabilitation 32*, 5, 717–724.

He, C. and Ma, H. (2017) Effectiveness of trigger point dry needling for plantar heel pain: A meta-analysis of seven randomized controlled trials. *Journal of Pain Research 10*, 1933–1942.

Hong, C.Z. (1994) Lidocaine injection versus dry needling to myofascial trigger point: The importance of the local twitch response. *American Journal of Physical Medicine and Rehabilitation 73*, 4, 256–263.

Hsieh, Y.L., Chou, L.W., Joe, Y.S. and Hong, C.Z. (2011) Spinal cord mechanism involving the remote effects of dry needling on the irritability of myofascial trigger spots in rabbit skeletal muscle. *Archives of Physical Medicine and Rehabilitation 92*, 7, 1098–1105.

Hsieh, Y.L., Kao, M.J., Kuan, T.S., Chen, S.M., Chen, J.T. and Hong, C.Z. (2007) Dry needling to a key myofascial trigger point may reduce the irritability of satellite MTrPs. *American Journal of Physical Medicine and Rehabilitation* 86, 5, 397–403.

Hsieh, Y.L., Yang, C.C., Liu, S.Y., Chou, L.W. and Hong, C.Z. (2014) Remote dose-dependent effects of dry needling at distant myofascial trigger spots of rabbit skeletal muscles on reduction of substance P levels of proximal muscle and spinal cords. *BioMed Research International 2014*, 982121.

Hsieh, Y.L., Yang, S.A., Yang, C.C. and Chou, L.W. (2012) Dry needling at myofascial trigger spots of rabbit skeletal muscles modulates the biochemicals associated with pain, inflammation, and hypoxia. *Evidence-Based Complementary and Alternative Medicine 2012*, 342165.

Kharazmi, A.S., Okhovatian, F., Baghban, A.A., Mosallanezhad, Z., Kojidi, M.M. and Azimi, H. (2020) Effects of dry needling on symptomatic hallux valgus: A randomized single blind clinical trial. *Journal of Bodywork and Movement Therapies* 24, 3, 246–251.

Kuan, T.S., Hsieh, Y.L., Chen, S.M., Chen, J.T., Yen, W.C. and Hong, C.Z. (2007) The myofascial trigger point region: Correlation between the degree of irritability and the prevalence of endplate noise. *American Journal of Physical Medicine and Rehabilitation* 86, 3, 183–189.

Lavelle, E.D., Lavelle, W. and Smith, H.S. (2007) Myofascial trigger points. *Anesthesiology Clinics* 25, 4, 841–851.

Leung, L. (2012) Neurophysiological basis of acupuncture-induced analgesia – an updated review. *Journal of Acupuncture and Meridian Studies* 5, 6, 261–270.

Liu, Q.G., Liu, L., Huang, Q.M., Nguyen, T.T., Ma, Y.T. and Zhao, J.M. (2017) Decreased spontaneous electrical activity and acetylcholine at myofascial trigger spots after dry needling treatment: A pilot study. *Evidence-Based Complementary and Alternative Medicine 2017*, 3938191.

López-González, L., Falla, D., Lázaro-Navas, I., Lorenzo-Sánchez-Aguilera, C. *et al.* (2021) Effects of dry needling on neuromuscular control of ankle stabilizer muscles and center of pressure displacement in basketball players with chronic ankle instability: A single-blinded randomized controlled trial. *International Journal of Environmental Research and Public Health* 18, 4, 2092.

Lundeberg, T. (2013) Mechanisms of Acupuncture in Pain: A Physiological Perspective in a Clinical Context. In H. Hong (ed.) *Acupuncture: Theories and Evidence*. World Scientific.

Méndez-Rebolledo, G., Guzmán-Muñoz, E., Gatica-Rojas, V. and Zbinden-Foncea, H. (2015) Longer reaction time of the fibularis longus muscle and reduced postural control in basketball players with functional ankle instability: A pilot study. *Physical Therapy in Sport* 16, 3, 242–247.

Mullins, J.F., Hoch, M.C., Kosik, K.B., Heebner, N.R. *et al.* (2021a) Effect of dry needling on spinal reflex excitability and postural control in individuals with chronic ankle instability. *Journal of Manipulative and Physiological Therapeutics* 44, 1, 25–34.

Mullins, J.F., Nitz, A.J. and Hoch, M.C. (2021b) Dry needling equilibration theory: A mechanistic explanation for enhancing sensorimotor function in individuals with chronic ankle instability. *Physiotherapy Theory and Practice* 37, 6, 672–681.

Niddam, D.M., Chan, R.C., Lee, S.H., Yeh, T.C. and Hsieh, J.C. (2007) Central modulation of pain evoked from myofascial trigger point. *The Clinical Journal of Pain* 23, 5, 440–448.

Perreault, T., Dunning, J. and Butts, R. (2017) The local twitch response during trigger point dry needling: Is it necessary for successful outcomes? *Journal of Bodywork and Movement Therapies* 21, 4, 940–947.

Pietrosimone, B.G. and Gribble, P.A. (2012) Chronic ankle instability and corticomotor excitability of the fibularis longus muscle. *Journal of Athletic Training* 47, 6, 621–626.

Rossi, A., Blaustein, S., Brown, J., Dieffenderfer, K. *et al.* (2017) Spinal and peripheral dry needling versus peripheral dry needling alone among individuals with a history of lateral ankle sprain: A randomized controlled trial. *International Journal of Sports Physical Therapy* 12, 7, 1034.

Salom-Moreno, J., Ayuso-Casado, B., Tamaral-Costa, B., Sánchez-Milá, Z., Fernández-de-Las-Peñas, C. and Alburquerque-Sendín, F. (2015) Trigger point dry needling and proprioceptive exercises for the management of chronic ankle instability: A randomized clinical trial. *Evidence-Based Complementary and Alternative Medicine* 2015, 790209.

Shah, J.P., Danoff, J.V., Desai, M.J., Parikh, S. *et al.* (2008) Biochemicals associated with pain and inflammation are elevated in sites near to and remote from active myofascial trigger points. *Archives of Physical Medicine and Rehabilitation* 89, 1, 16–23.

Shah, J.P., Phillips, T., Danoff, J.V. and Gerber, L.H. (2003) A novel microanalytical technique for assaying soft tissue demonstrates significant quantitative biochemical differences in 3 clinically distinct groups: normal, latent, and active. *Archives of Physical Medicine and Rehabilitation* 84, 9, E4.

Srbely, J.Z., Dickey, J.P., Lee, D. and Lowerison, M. (2010) Dry needle stimulation of myofascial trigger points evokes segmental anti-nociceptive effects. *Journal of Rehabilitation Medicine* 42, 5, 463–468.

Staud, R. and Price, D.D. (2006) Mechanisms of acupuncture analgesia for clinical and experimental pain. *Expert Review of Neurotherapeutics* 6, 5, 661–667.

Tsai, C.T., Hsieh, L.F., Kuan, T.S., Kao, M.J., Chou, L.W. and Hong, C.Z. (2010) Remote effects of dry needling on the irritability of the myofascial trigger point in the upper trapezius muscle. *American Journal of Physical Medicine & Rehabilitation* 89, 2, 133–140.

Ying, J., Xu, Y., István, B. and Ren, F. (2021) Adjusted indirect and mixed comparisons of conservative treatments for hallux valgus: A systematic review and network meta-analysis. *International Journal of Environmental Research and Public Health* 18, 7, 3841.

Chapter 12

Muscle Energy Techniques for the Foot and Ankle

Muscle energy techniques (MET) are safe, effective and non-invasive treatment techniques suitable for a variety of musculoskeletal conditions. MET can be used to treat somatic dysfunction, restore joint range of motion (ROM), support a weakened muscle, release muscular tension, temporarily lengthen a shortened or contracted muscle, improve blood circulation and lymphatic flow, and reduce musculoskeletal pain (Thomas *et al.*, 2019; Waxenbaum and Lu, 2020; Ahmed *et al.*, 2021). Historically, it was first developed in 1948 by an osteopathic physician, Fred Mitchell (Sr.), after he was inspired by the work of a fellow osteopath, T.J. Ruddy. Mitchell's son, Fred Mitchell (Jr.), and a Czech physician, Karel Lewit, later made a major contribution to the refinements and standardisation of MET methods (Goodridge, 1981; Lewit and Simons, 1984; Fryer, 2011). However, that is not the end of MET evolution. It has continued to evolve over the years under practitioners from various body and movement therapy professions.

Today there are different MET protocols with varied paradigms and specifics, which differ in the frequency of repetitions, duration of rest, contraction and stretch phases, and strength of contraction (Fryer and Ruszkowski, 2004; Lari *et al.*, 2016; Waxenbaum and Lu, 2020). MET protocols suggested by Greenman (2003) and Chaitow and Crenshaw (2006) are currently two of the most prominent of all application methods. The Greenman method involves 3–5 repetitions with a 5–7-second resting phase to release tissue tension in the targeted area. On the other hand, the Chaitow method applies four repetitions with a 30–60-second relaxation phase after each contraction. However, it is yet to be determined which protocol is more effective.

As discussed above, MET has evolved out of osteopathic medicine; however, it is now practised by health professionals from various disciplines including physiotherapists, chiropractors, massage therapists, manual therapists as well as allopathic physicians (Chaitow and Crenshaw, 2006). The growing popularity of MET among clinicians can be attributed to its pain-modulatory and ROM-improving effects. Although there is limited evidence supporting the application of MET typologies for foot or ankle conditions, an apparent consensus has been reached on its beneficial effects in other circumstances, particularly low back pain (Franke *et al.*, 2015; Sbardella *et al.*, 2021). This chapter provides a general overview of MET – in particular, what it is, how it works, its mode of application and general contraindications.

What is MET?

MET is a form of soft-tissue osteopathic technique that involves a patient-initiated voluntary contraction of skeletal muscle against a therapist-applied counterforce in a precise direction and position. MET protocols are unique in osteopathic medicine, as they are active manipulation or mobilisation techniques in which both the therapist and the patient are actively involved. During a MET procedure, the patient first undergoes a resistive force against their voluntary isometric contractions, which is then followed by assisted stretching (Chaitow and Crenshaw, 2006; DeStefano, 2011; Fryer, 2011).

MET is technically somewhat comparable to the advanced stretching technique called proprioceptive neuromuscular facilitation (PNF) (Thomas *et al.*, 2018). However, the major difference between MET and PNF is that MET primarily aims to activate tonic muscle fibres and thus applies comparatively lower forces than those of PNF. In contrast, PNF mainly recruits phasic muscle fibres, which are generally activated when considerably greater forces are applied (about 25% of an individual's maximal force) (Ptaszkowski *et al.*, 2015; Thomas *et al.*, 2019).

General principles

MET primarily aims to relax the muscle or muscle group by reducing hypertonicity, which is thought to be the source of pain, functional impairment or somatic dysfunction in a body part and/or joint. Two general principles are thought to be involved in the relaxation of muscles with MET: autogenic inhibition and reciprocal inhibition. Both of these phenomena are known to involve Golgi tendon organs (GTOs) and the muscle spindles to induce neurophysiological responses (Chaitow and Crenshaw, 2006; Waxenbaum and Lu, 2020).

Autogenic inhibition

The GTOs are mechanoreceptors responsible for sensing increased tension when a muscle is exposed to contractile force. When GTOs sense a muscle contraction or stretching, they respond by activating type Ib afferent fibres, which consequently cause a synaptic activation of the Ib inhibitory interneurons (Laporte and Lloyd, 1952; Gordon, 2007). These interneurons then send 'inhibitory' input to the efferent α-motor neurons. As a result, an inhibitory, negative feedback is sent from the brain to inhibit the excitability of the stretched muscle and allow the contraction of the antagonist muscle. This sudden relaxation of the muscle is known as the autogenic inhibition reflex or the inverse myotatic reflex (Sharman *et al.*, 2006; Hindle *et al.*, 2012).

Reciprocal inhibition

Muscle spindles are mechanoreceptors sensitive to stretching. When a muscle fibre is stretched, it activates the stretch reflex through activation of the Ia muscle spindle afferents. These afferents stimulate the α- and γ-motor neurons of the same (homonymous) muscle and ultimately cause it to contract. Simultaneously, another branch of the Ia afferents innervates the inhibitory interneurons, which in turn synapse on to the α-motor neurons of the opposing muscle. The innervation by the inhibitory interneurons eventually inhibits the α-motor neurons from activating and thus leads to a relaxation in the antagonist muscle. This phenomenon is commonly known as reciprocal inhibition (Petersen *et al.*, 1999; Rowlands *et al.*, 2003; Waxenbaum and Lu, 2020).

Types of MET

Autogenic inhibition MET

There are currently two types of MET based on the principles of autogenic inhibition:

- post-isometric relaxation

- post-facilitation stretching.

Post-isometric relaxation (**PIR**) is the best-known MET typology based on the autogenic inhibition concept. As discussed above, PIR is the physiological response induced by GTOs following an isometric contraction of a muscle. Shortly after an isometric contraction, a muscle, or group, is assumed to experience an effect of reduced tonicity due to the activation of the Ib inhibitory interneurons, which eventually leads to a sudden relaxation of the muscle. This assumed effect is known as PIR (Lewit and Simons, 1984; Chaitow and Crenshaw, 2006). The reduction in tone means that the reflexive components of the isometric contraction are reduced. These effects ultimately relax a hypertonic muscle, encourage joint ROM and increase muscle length (Ferber *et al.*, 2002; Rowlands *et al.*, 2003).

Post-facilitation stretching (**PFS**), developed by Dr Vladimir Janda, is another MET typology that follows the principles of autogenic inhibition (Page *et al.*, 2011). PFS involves a maximal contraction of the muscle followed by a rapid stretching to a new barrier. From the technical standpoint, PFS is a more aggressive form of autogenic MET than PIR, and thus more beneficial for the shortened muscles (Page, 2012).

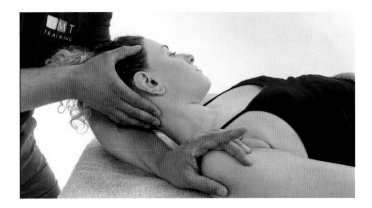

Reciprocal inhibition MET

Reciprocal inhibition MET follows the principles of reciprocal inhibition described above. It involves a voluntary contraction of the agonist muscle followed by passive stretching of the antagonist muscle (Thomas *et al.*, 2019). When the isometric contraction of the agonist occurs, the antagonist is reciprocally inhibited or deactivated. This reduces hypertonicity in the antagonist muscle and ultimately leads to its relaxation and lengthening. This phenomenon can therefore be helpful in achieving an added potential of introducing further ROM and a degree of ease to the affected joint (Crone, 1993; Chaitow and Crenshaw, 2006).

Physiologic mechanisms

As discussed above, proponents of MET primarily take advantage of the principal mechanisms of autogenic and reciprocal inhibitions to explain its therapeutic effects. However, studies evaluating the effects of pre-isometric contraction on joint extensibility have reported an increase in joint ROM but no changes in resting electromyographic (EMG) activity (Magnusson *et al.*, 1996; Thomas *et al.*, 2019). Some studies, on the other hand, noted alterations in EMG activity during eccentrically and concentrically loaded isometric contractions (Christova and Kossev, 2000; Garner *et al.*, 2008). Hence, there is still no consensus regarding the exact mechanisms through which MET exerts its therapeutic effects.

Various theories have been proposed, including changes in joint proprioception, motor programming and viscoelastic properties (Ballantyne *et al.*, 2003; Fryer, 2011). It has been hypothesised that MET-induced stimulation of GTOs and muscle spindles activates joint proprioceptors and mechanoreceptors, which in turn alter the motor programming and control of the target joint, and eventually activate the descending pain-inhibitory pathways. On the other hand, MET is known to alter the viscoelastic properties of the soft tissue, which may have an effect on joint ROM and pain modulation (Skyba *et al.*, 2003; Thomas *et al.*, 2019). The reduction in muscle tone with MET may be attributed to the stimulation of fascia and the increase in local vasodilation (Schleip, 2003). In addition, the application of MET is shown to increase stretch tolerance, which has been thought to play a role in the increased flexibility of the muscles, or their group (Ballantyne *et al.*, 2003; Thomas *et al.*, 2018). In summary, only a limited number of studies have so far investigated the possible physiological mechanisms of MET, and thus more research is needed to establish these hypotheses.

Contraindications to MET

MET is contraindicated in certain patient populations. Because MET is an active technique and requires full cooperation from the patient, it is contraindicated for those who will be unable to bear the added exertion or actively cooperate during the application (Lafans and Troncoso, 2021).

The following conditions should be considered contraindications to MET:

- poor energy
- significant joint disease
- recent surgery
- fractures
- severe osteoporosis
- ligamentous laxity
- deep vein thrombosis or thrombophlebitis
- avulsion injuries
- haemorrhagic conditions
- impaired bone, tendon, ligament or joint integrity
- cardiac failure
- damaged or at-risk skin
- open wounds
- metastatic cancer
- active infection.

In addition, if the therapist suspects any pathology, MET should not be applied until a correct diagnosis is made. MET is applicable in the presence of certain pathologies (e.g. osteoporosis, arthritis), but an accurate diagnosis of the presenting condition is needed to modify the dosage of application such as the frequency of repetitions, duration of rest, force of contraction, amount of stretching and amount of effort used.

MET can be a useful addition to the treatment of foot and ankle conditions and complement structural techniques such as mobilisation and manipulation. Here is a selection of foot and ankle MET techniques.

MET techniques for the lower extremities

Rectus femoris
Rectus femoris – supine – Thomas position

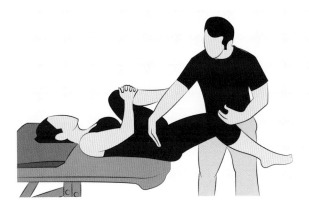

- An alternative MET for the rectus femoris is based on the modified Thomas test position.

- The patient adopts the position of the modified Thomas test as shown.

- You control the position of the patient's hip and passively flex their knee, slowly, towards their glute.

- Locate the first barrier.

- From the first barrier, the patient is asked to extend the knee against resistance.

- After the ten-second contraction and in the relaxation phase, passively take the knee into further flexion.

Keynote

- This can be quite intense for the patient, so proceed slowly.

- If the patient has lumbar pathology, take your time or change to an alternative.

Rectus femoris – prone – PIR

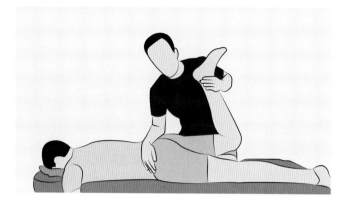

- The patient is in the prone position, the therapist is on the ipsilateral side. The leg is placed on the therapist's knee and the therapist passively flexes the patient's right knee until the first barrier is assessed.

- From the barrier position, the patient is asked to extend their knee against a resistance applied by the therapist.

- After a ten-second contraction and in the relaxation phase, the therapist encourages the knee into further flexion.

- After the contraction and in the relaxation phase, the therapist controls the knee and slowly flexes the knee and hip at the same time.

- This will induce a lengthening at the origin and at the insertion of the rectus femoris.

Keynote

- If the patient cannot feel the stretch near the insertion, you could add hip extension.

Tensor fasciae latae

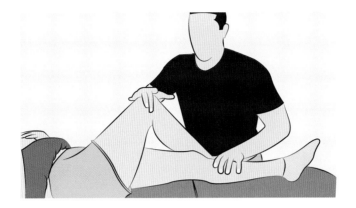

Tensor fasciae latae (TFL) – supine – PIR

- The patient is in the supine position.

- Cross the patient's flexed leg over the leg you will be treating.

- The therapist controls the patient's flexed knee with their hand and holds on to the patient's lateral malleolus.

- Adduct the leg until the first barrier is felt.

- From the first barrier, the patient is asked to abduct their leg against resistance applied.

- After a ten-second contraction and in the relaxation phase, the therapist passively takes the patient's leg into further adduction.

- This will lengthen the right TFL.

Keynote

- If the patient has a knee pathology, you may need to hold the lateral aspect of the knee rather than the ankle to avoid stress.

- You can use a mobilisation belt to restrict movement of the hip.

- The patient will need to hold the table to avoid unnecessary movement.

Hamstrings

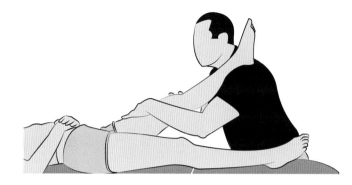

Hamstring – supine – PIR – non-specific technique

- This technique is for lengthening the hamstrings as a group.

- The therapist adopts a standing posture and passively controls the patient's right leg into hip flexion until a barrier is felt in the hamstrings group.

- Once the barrier is felt, reduce hip flexion by up to 5°.

- From this position, the patient's lower leg is placed on your shoulder.

- The patient is asked to push down against the shoulder of the therapist for ten seconds.

- After the contraction of the hamstrings and in the relaxation phase, the therapist passively takes the right leg into further hip flexion.

Keynote

- Place a towel over your shoulder to give added comfort to both you and the patient.

- Make sure the patient uses limited power on this technique.

Adductors

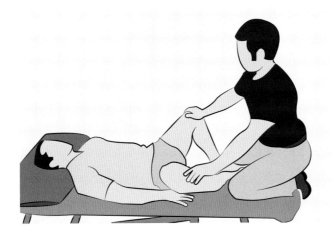

Adductors – supine – PIR

- The patient is in the supine position with their knees bent and their calcaneus together.

- This technique aims to target:

  - adductor brevis

  - adductor longus

  - adductor magnus.

- The patient's hips are passively taken into abduction by the therapist until the first barrier is felt.

- From the barrier, the patient is asked to adduct their hips against resistance applied by the therapist.

- After a ten-second contraction and in the relaxation phase, the hips are then passively taken into further abduction by the control of the therapist.

Keynote

- You can perform this technique either unilaterally or bilaterally.

- Limit the amount of power used, especially with patients who have a history of pubic symphysis pathology or pelvic floor dysfunction.

Gastrocnemius

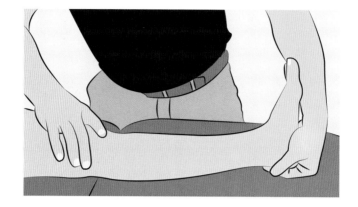

Gastrocnemius – supine – PIR

- The patient is in the supine position.

- Hold the calcaneus from the plantar aspect with your forearm on the ball of the foot.

- The patient is asked to push their toes away (plantarflexion) to activate the gastrocnemius on to your arm for ten seconds.

- After a ten-second contraction and in the relaxation phase, the therapist encourages dorsiflexion to promote lengthening of the gastrocnemius.

Keynote

- Make sure the patient does not use full force here.

- The patient needs to control their breathing to maintain contraction control.

Soleus

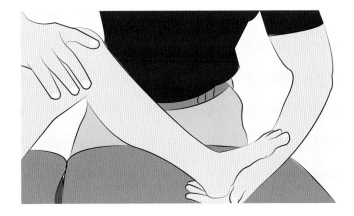

Soleus – supine – PIR

- The patient is in the supine position.

- The knee is in slight flexion, to increase the bias towards the soleus.

- The therapist controls the position of the lower limb and ankle by holding on to the calcaneus from the plantar aspect.

- From this position, the therapist slowly encourages dorsiflexion of the ankle until the first barrier is felt.

- From the barrier, the patient is asked to plantarflex the ankle to activate the contraction.

- After a ten-second contraction and in the relaxation phase, the therapist gently encourages the ankle into further dorsiflexion to the next barrier.

Keynote

- Make sure the patient does not use full force here.

- The patient needs to control their breathing to maintain contraction control.

References

Ahmed, U.A., Nadasan, T., Van Oosterwijck, J. and Maharaj, S.S. (2021) The effect of muscles energy technique in the management of chronic mechanical low back pain: A scoping review. *Journal of Back and Musculoskeletal Rehabilitation 34*, 2, 179–193.

Ballantyne, F., Fryer, G. and McLaughlin, P. (2003) The effect of muscle energy technique on hamstring extensibility: The mechanism of altered flexibility. *Journal of Osteopathic Medicine 6*, 2, 59–63.

Chaitow, L. and Crenshaw, K. (2006) *Muscle Energy Techniques*. Elsevier Health Sciences.

Christova, P. and Kossev, A. (2000) Human motor unit activity during concentric and eccentric movements. *Electromyography and Clinical Neurophysiology 40*, 6, 331–338.

Crone, C. (1993) Reciprocal inhibition in man. *Danish Medical Bulletin 40*, 5, 571–581.

DeStefano, L.A. (2011) *Greenman's Principles of Manual Medicine*. Lippincott Williams & Wilkins.

Ferber, R., Osternig, L.R. and Gravelle, D.C. (2002) Effect of PNF stretch techniques on knee flexor muscle EMG activity in older adults. *Journal of Electromyography and Kinesiology 12*, 5, 391–397.

Franke, H., Fryer, G., Ostelo, R.W. and Kamper, S.J. (2015) Muscle energy technique for non-specific low-back pain. *Cochrane Database of Systematic Reviews 2015*, 2, CD009852.

Fryer, G. (2011) Muscle energy technique: An evidence-informed approach. *International Journal of Osteopathic Medicine 14*, 1, 3–9.

Fryer, G. and Ruszkowski, W. (2004) The influence of contraction duration in muscle energy technique applied to the atlanto-axial joint. *Journal of Osteopathic Medicine 7*, 2, 79–84.

Garner, J.C., Blackburn, T., Weimar, W. and Campbell, B. (2008) Comparison of electromyographic activity during eccentrically versus concentrically loaded isometric contractions. *Journal of Electromyography and Kinesiology 18*, 3, 466–471.

Goodridge, J.P. (1981) Muscle energy technique: Definition, explanation, methods of procedure. *The Journal of the American Osteopathic Association 81*, 12, 67–74.

Gordon, C. (2007) Do Golgi tendon organs really inhibit muscle activity at high force levels to save muscles from injury, and adapt with strength training? *Sports Biomechanics 1*, 2, 239–349.

Greenman, P.E. (2003) *Principles of Manual Medicine*. Lippincott Williams & Wilkins.

Hindle, K., Whitcomb, T., Briggs, W. and Hong, J. (2012) Proprioceptive neuromuscular facilitation (PNF): Its mechanisms and effects on range of motion and muscular function. *Journal of Human Kinetics 31*, 105–113.

Lafans, K. and Troncoso, V. (2021) Osteopathic Manipulative Treatment: Muscle Energy Procedure-Lumbar Vertebrae. StatPearls [Internet], www.ncbi.nlm.nih.gov/books/NBK560895

Laporte, Y. and Lloyd, D.P. (1952) Nature and significance of the reflex connections established by large afferent fibers of muscular origin. *American Journal of Physiology 169*, 3, 609–621.

Lari, A.Y., Okhovatian, F., Sadat Naimi, S. and Baghban, A.A. (2016) The effect of the combination of dry needling and MET on latent trigger point upper trapezius in females. *Manual Therapy 21*, 204–209.

Lewit, K. and Simons, D.G. (1984) Myofascial pain: Relief by post-isometric relaxation. *Archives of Physical Medicine and Rehabilitation 65*, 8, 452–456.

Magnusson, S.P., Simonsen, E.B., Aagaard, P., Dyhre-Poulsen, P., McHugh, M.P. and Kjaer, M. (1996) Mechanical and physiological responses to stretching with and without preisometric contraction in human skeletal muscle. *Archives of Physical Medicine and Rehabilitation 77*, 4, 373–378.

Page, P. (2012) Current concepts in muscle stretching for exercise and rehabilitation. *International Journal of Sports Physical Therapy 7*, 1, 109–119.

Page, P., Frank, C. and Lardner, R. (2011) Assessment and treatment of muscle imbalance: The Janda approach. *Journal of Orthopedic and Sports Physical Therapy 41*, 10, 799–800.

Petersen, N., Morita, H. and Nielsen, J. (1999) Modulation of reciprocal inhibition between ankle extensors and flexors during walking in man. *The Journal of Physiology 520*, 2, 605–619.

Ptaszkowski, K., Slupska, L., Paprocka-Borowicz, M., Kołcz-Trzęsicka, A. *et al.* (2015) Comparison of the short-term outcomes after postisometric muscle relaxation or Kinesio taping application for normalization of the upper trapezius muscle tone and the pain relief: A preliminary study. *Evidence-Based Complementary and Alternative Medicine 2015*, 721938.

Rowlands, A.V., Marginson, V.F. and Lee, J. (2003) Chronic flexibility gains: Effect of isometric contraction duration during proprioceptive neuromuscular facilitation stretching techniques. *Research Quarterly for Exercise and Sport 74*, 1, 47–51.

Sbardella, S., La Russa, C., Bernetti, A., Mangone, M. *et al.* (2021) Muscle energy technique in the rehabilitative treatment for acute and chronic non-specific neck pain: A systematic review. *Healthcare 9*, 6, 746.

Schleip, R. (2003) Fascial plasticity – a new neurobiological explanation: Part 2. *Journal of Bodywork and Movement Therapies 7*, 2, 104–116.

Sharman, M.J., Cresswell, A.G. and Riek, S. (2006) Proprioceptive neuromuscular facilitation stretching. *Sports Medicine 36*, 11, 929–939.

Skyba, D.A., Radhakrishnan, R., Rohlwing, J.J., Wright, A. and Sluka, K.A. (2003) Joint manipulation reduces hyperalgesia by activation of monoamine receptors but not opioid or GABA receptors in the spinal cord. *Pain 106*, 1–2, 159–168.

Thomas, E., Bianco, A., Paoli, A. and Palma, A. (2018) The relation between stretching typology and stretching duration: The effects on range of motion. *International Journal of Sports Medicine 39*, 4, 243–254.

Thomas, E., Cavallaro, A.R., Mani, D., Bianco, A. and Palma, A. (2019) The efficacy of muscle energy techniques in symptomatic and asymptomatic subjects: A systematic review. *Chiropractic and Manual Therapies 27*, 1, 1–18.

Waxenbaum, J.A. and Lu, M. (2020) Physiology, Muscle Energy. StatPearls [Internet], www.ncbi.nlm.nih.gov/books/NBK559029

Chapter 13

Sports Taping and Strapping

IAIN BARROWMAN

The use of taping or strapping as a therapeutic tool has increased greatly in recent years, particularly after the 2008 and 2012 Olympics. The increased globalisation of healthcare products has also played a role in the growing popularity of this therapeutic technique (Grant *et al.*, 2014). Today it is frequently used by rehabilitation clinicians from various healthcare professions (e.g. sports medicine physicians, physical therapists, osteopaths, athletic trainers and chiropractors) as an aid to prevent and treat many musculoskeletal conditions. Therapy tape, however, has been in use for well over 100 years. In the literature, the first recorded evidence of its effects could be traced back to 1969 (Simon, 1969). In the early days, medical doctors primarily utilised the taping technique to keep unstable joints in position; however, much has changed since it was first used (Bandyopadhyay and Mahapatra, 2012).

Historically, rigid tapes made of rubber adhesive were the first to be used as a therapeutic tool to limit or restrict the movement of joints. These tapes, however, were later found to be irritable to the skin; thus, newer versions of these tapes were introduced over the years with improved materials (Baquie, 2002; Bandyopadhyay and Mahapatra, 2012). In addition to the traditional athletic tapes, today there are various types of tapes with varied materials in common use including kinesiology tape, Mulligan tape and McConnell tape, to name a few (Polakowski, 2015). Some variations of these tapes are made of highly flexible and stretchy materials, which allow the wearer a full range of motion, while others made from rigid materials are primarily used to support or protect injured joints while in play. Proponents of these tapes claim that their usage can prevent injuries, stabilise joint movement, reduce pain and swelling, increase proprioception, improve blood flow, optimise athletic performance and improve physical activity. However, evidence to support these claims is still very limited (Dizon and Reyes, 2010; Zwiers *et al.*, 2016; Trofa *et al.*, 2020; Nunes *et al.*, 2021).

Kinesiology tape or Kinesio tape (KT) is currently the most popular taping method in use. It was heavily featured in the 2008 and 2012 Olympics and gained overnight popularity among athletes and laypeople (Trofa *et al.*, 2020). However, KT is actually an umbrella term, which includes a variety of elastic adhesive tapes that differ very subtly in their physical properties (Kase *et al.*, 2003). Although there are several KT brands, the proposed therapeutic effects have been similar. Proposed mechanical and physiological effects of KT include the facilitation of joint movement and muscle realignment and an improvement in various physical parameters, including pain levels, lymphatic return and muscle strength (Wilkerson, 2002; Zwiers *et al.*, 2016; Shin *et al.*, 2020; Nunes *et al.*, 2021). In addition, KT is probably the most studied of all taping methods. In fact, the number of scholarly publications on this taping technique has increased greatly in recent years. Nevertheless, the clinical efficacy of KT has remained debatable (Slevin *et al.*, 2020; Nunes *et al.*, 2021).

This chapter gives a general overview of traditional athletic taping and KT – what they are and their proposed mechanism of action. We will also describe their clinical relevance in the treatment of ankle and foot conditions.

Athletic taping techniques

What are traditional athletic tapes?

Traditional athletic tapes primarily include non-elastic, white sports tape. These have been in use for many, many years. A common example of these tapes is the rigid zinc oxide tape, which is a non-elastic, rayon-cotton strapping tape coated with a strong zinc oxide-based adhesive.

Rigid zinc oxide tapes do not stretch vertically or horizontally and mainly aim to restrict movement of the joint. For example, they can be used for securing the ankle or restricting the motion of injured joint(s) during a sports activity. However, as these tapes tightly wrap around joints, they must be used for only short periods. Their prolonged use can cause problems with blood and lymphatic circulation. In summary, these tapes are mainly used as a means for the prophylaxis and rehabilitation of anatomical structures involved in the injury (Hughes and McLean, 1988; Birrer and Poole, 2004; Bandyopadhyay and Mahapatra, 2012).

Other types of athletic tape are often used along with the zinc oxide tape, including the tear elastic adhesive bandage (EAB), non-tear EAB, fixation tape, underwrap tape, cohesive tape, etc. Table 13.1 summarises the clinical characteristics of these tapes.

Table 13.1 Characteristics of various types of athletic tape

Tape name	Characteristics	Available size
Tear EAB	A special type of EAB that can be easily torn by hand and manipulated around fingers Often used as a covering or underlay when securing white or tan zinc oxide strappings Its fabric is more versatile than the non-tear EAB and allows light support and compression for lymphatic flow	25 mm, 50 mm, 75 mm
Non-tear EAB	Heavier, thicker, much stronger and less breathable than tear EAB Includes latex-free, woven cotton with a zinc oxide adhesive Often used as a halfway point between zinc oxide white and tear EAB Can stretch up to 125–140% of its length Good for non-weight-bearing joints as it gives some support with flexibility Requires scissors to cut it	25 mm, 50 mm, 75 mm
Cohesive bandage	An on-the-go sports tape that is highly flexible, hand-tearable, easy-to-apply and lightweight Can be applied with varying degrees of tension and pressure Allows reapplication and adjustment multiple times Can be applied over wounds, sprains and strains as a compression Secures heat packs, dressings, grip socks and shin pads in place	25 mm, 50 mm, 75 mm, 100 mm
Fixation tape	A rigid, non-woven, adhesive tape commonly known by its brand name, Hypafix® Used widely for dressing retention or fixation Can be used as a protective barrier between the skin and the more aggressive adhesives (e.g. zinc oxide tape) Smaller strips of this tape can be utilised as anchors to help the zinc oxide tape stay in place	50 mm, 100 mm, 150 mm
Underwrap tape	Made from a lightweight foam that is porous, water-repellent and easy to use Usually acts as a thin barrier to protect the skin from the irritation of wearing adhesive zinc oxide tapes or cohesive elastic bandages Sticks to adhesive tapes perfectly and prevents slippage during use or exposure to sweat Makes taping and strapping with adhesive tapes more comfortable and longer lasting	50 mm, 70 mm

Mechanism of action of athletic tapes

The exact mechanism(s) underlying the beneficial effects of athletic tapes is not fully understood. It has been suggested that a combination of mechanisms is involved in the observed therapeutic effects of these tapes. One of the frequently proposed theories is based on the mechanical aspect of taping. This theory proposes that taping provides mechanical support to the injured anatomic structures by restricting abnormal movement (Zwiers *et al.*, 2016).

Studies conducted to evaluate this theory have also supported the effectiveness of athletic tapes in limiting the range of motion to some extent (Trégouët *et al.*, 2013). In fact, an early comparative study by Bunch *et al.* (1985) reported that the best level of ankle support was achieved with fresh adhesive tape. Adhesive taping was also found to be superior to bracing in limiting maximal ankle dorsiflexion (Cordova *et al.*, 2002). In addition, a randomised trial by Lardenoye *et al.* (2012) demonstrated the same degree of restriction in ankle ROM with both semi-rigid brace and inelastic tape. Rigid tapes were also found to decrease the inversion velocity and reduce the time to maximum inversion (Riemann *et al.*, 2002). It is suggested that the reduction in inversion velocity by taping affords the peroneal muscle extra time to respond (Zwiers *et al.*, 2016). However, a major downside of using these tapes is that they often lose their restrictive qualities during exercise or athletic activity. Rigid taping is known to achieve about 50% of restriction in ROM, of which only 10% remains after 20 minutes of exercise (Greene and Hillman, 1990; Forbes *et al.*, 2013; Best *et al.*, 2014). This makes the mechanical theory of preventive mechanism questionable, as only a small percentage of restrictive effect is achievable with rigid adhesive taping during athletic activity.

Other proposed theories of the beneficial effects of athletic tapes primarily focus on the neuromuscular aspects. It is presumed that the use of adhesive taping increases proprioceptive input to the brain by stimulating cutaneous mechanoreceptors, which in turn influences postural stability and peroneal muscle latency and reflexes. The substantial role of cutaneous mechanoreceptors is also supported in a study by Stecco *et al.* (2008), where the authors noted that the fascial layers closer to the skin have a denser population of mechanoreceptors compared with the layers deeper in the tissues. However, so far there is not much evidence to support the effects of taping on joint proprioception. In fact, a systematic review by Raymond *et al.* (2012) found no conclusive evidence in support of the proprioceptive input theory of athletic taping. From the available evidence, it seems that the therapeutic effect of taping on proprioception diminishes during exercise or athletic activity, and its preventive usage is more beneficial after first-time ankle or foot injury (Lohrer *et al.*, 1999; Raymond *et al.*, 2012; Zwiers *et al.*, 2016).

On the other hand, the effects of taping on peroneal longus muscle activity and latency have been studied extensively. However, there is no high-quality evidence that inelastic athletic taping of the ankle shortens the reaction time or changes the activity of the peroneal muscle (Lohrer *et al.*, 1999; Briem *et al.*, 2011; Trégouët *et al.*, 2013; Yoon *et al.*, 2013; Juchler *et al.*, 2016). The results of its effects on muscle latency are also conflicting (Shima *et al.*, 2005; Kelly *et al.*, 2010; Knight and Weimar, 2011). In addition, studies on the effect of taping on postural control have also found no plausible evidence of improvement or changes in stabilometric values (Cordova *et al.*, 2005; De Ridder *et al.*, 2015; Inglés *et al.*, 2019; Yin and Wang, 2020). However, there is a high likelihood that the use of taping has a psychological effect. In fact, several studies have described a placebo effect of athletic taping. Patients were reported to be more confident, stable and reassured while having their ankle supported with taping compared with no tape in performing functional or sport-specific tasks (Olmsted *et al.*, 2004; Sawkins *et al.*, 2007; Delahunt *et al.*, 2010; Simon and Donahue, 2013; Yin and Wang, 2020). We believe this may be due to the feeling of support when they apply the tape.

What is KT?

KT, also known as tension taping, is a special form of therapeutic tape that offers an elastic alternative to the traditional rigid taping techniques. A Japanese chiropractor named Dr Kenso Kase first developed KT in the 1970s to overcome the problems of rigid athletic tapes. It characteristically differs from the traditional white tapes with its bright colours, wave-like grain design and water resistance and breathability properties. KT also sticks better to skin and can be worn for longer periods than the traditional tapes.

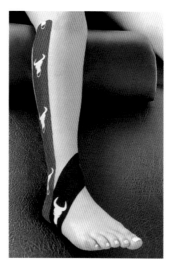

Clinicians usually apply KT over or around the edges of injured areas based on the understanding of joint movements and myofascial lines. From a functional standpoint, it mimics the elasticity of the skin and applies a pulling force to the skin. It is known to stretch up to 120–160% of its original length during application, after which it recoils to its normal length, providing a tensile force to the skin. This force is thought to provide therapeutic benefits by lifting the fascia and soft tissue and thereby facilitating the mobility of blood and lymphatic flow (Chang *et al.*, 2010).

How KT works

The underlying mechanisms through which KT works are still unclear. Proponents of KT have claimed numerous physiological effects based on several theories. There is a long-held notion that the mechanical properties of this taping technique influence fascia through neurosensory stimulation, which alters the neural input to the brain. As described above, Stecco *et al.* (2008) have already confirmed the presence of a greater density of mechanoreceptors in fascial layers. However, it is not yet known how KT provides its therapeutic effects influencing fascial mechanoreceptors.

Pamuk and Yucesoy (2015) studied the mechanical tissue changes following the application of kinesiology taping. They performed a magnetic resonance imaging (MRI) analysis before and after the taping application. The results affirmed their hypothesis that fascia in the whole limb experiences heterogenous deformations. Tu *et al.* (2016) conducted an observational study of changes to fascia in asymptotic individuals. It was noted that kinesiology taping could reduce the thoracolumbar fascial thickness and movement. These two studies do report the changes to fascia, but it is not clear how this is related to the reduction in pain or improvement in movement.

The proposed physiological effects of KT include the following:

- improving proprioceptive signals to the brain
- assisting in the repair of ligament or tendon damage
- increasing the flow of blood and lymph
- adjusting the misalignment of joints, muscles and myofascia
- diminishing input from afferent nerve fibres
- reducing pressure on subcutaneous nociceptors.

However, despite the growing popularity of KT among clinicians and athletes, there is conflicting evidence regarding its efficacy in the prevention and management of foot and ankle pathologies. Although there are not many high-quality studies, a number of systemic reviews have been published to date. These reviews, however, vary in their conclusions. Some reviews have reported little to no long-term benefit of KT for ankle or other musculoskeletal injuries compared with usual care or sham tape (Bassett *et al.*, 2010; Mostafavifar *et al.*, 2012; Morris *et al.*, 2013; Parreira *et al.*, 2014), while others reported an immediate reduction in pain, moderate improvements in movement and muscle activity, and positive effects on proprioception (Williams *et al.*, 2012; Kalron and Bar-Sela, 2013; Lim and Tay, 2015; Wilson and Bialocerkowski, 2015; Wang *et al.*, 2018).

There may be several reasons for the conflicting conclusions in these reviews, including lack of adequate power in the included studies, insufficient volume of evidence, inconsistency in the eligibility criteria, exclusion of relevant studies and inappropriate approach to the meta-analyses conducted. Recently, after evaluating 84 studies with meta-analysis, Nunes *et al.* (2021) concluded that current evidence neither supports nor encourages KT usage for the improvement of ankle function. The authors suggested that KT should be regarded as an aid to conventional treatments like other athletic taping techniques. They also emphasised that further research needs to be carried out to determine the efficacy of KT as an adjunctive technique.

Contraindications

In general, the contraindications for taping and strapping are similar to any form of manual therapy. They mainly include the following:

- sites of acute infection
- open wounds
- allergy to taping materials
- active cancer
- signs of serious trauma in the applicable area
- deep vein thrombosis
- signs of circulatory compromise in the applicable area
- fragile skin
- presence of skin conditions (e.g. eczema, psoriasis, tinea pedis)
- systemic diseases (e.g. diabetes, kidney disease, heart conditions)
- pregnancy.

Basic rigid foot and ankle strapping techniques
Sprained ankle

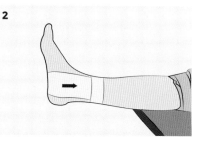

1

Start by wrapping a piece of tape around the leg 5 cm above the ankle bones. This will serve as a landmark.

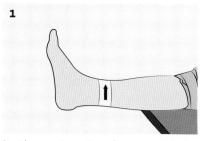

2

Using three pieces of overlapping tape, apply three stirrups. Centre the first piece of tape over the ankle bones. Secure all three with another landmark piece.

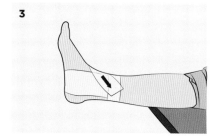

3

Using three pieces of overlapping tape, apply three Js. Start on the uninjured side.

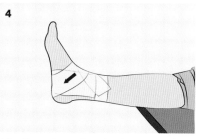

4

Using three pieces of overlapping tape, apply three figure-of-eights. Start on the uninjured side and end under the arch of the foot.

Simple arch support

Purpose: to support the arch and midfoot.

1 Apply anchor; secure under the fifth metatarsal and apply slight tension in an upward direction.

2 Apply additional strips moving from the distal to proximal aspect of the foot.

3 Use arch pad for additional support.

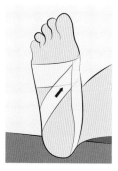
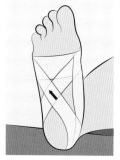
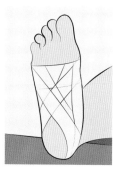

Alternative arch support

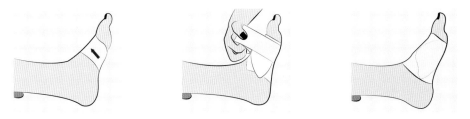

Achilles tendon strain

Purpose: to limit excessive dorsiflexion to reduce tension placed on the tendon.

1 Patient prone; foot in slight plantarflexion.
2 Place lubricated pad over Achilles tendon.
3 Apply anchors using non-elastic tape at the base of the metatarsals and 10–15 cm above the ankle.

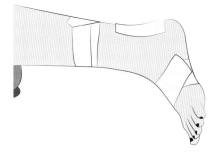

4 Apply 3–5 strips of non-elastic tape in an X pattern from distal to proximal anchor; this forms a check rein.
5 Re-anchor the X distally and proximally with non-elastic tape.
6 Patient moves to a seated position.
7 Apply a figure-of-eight and heel locks using non-elastic tape.

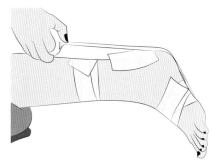

Shin splints taping

Purpose: to provide some relief of anterior shin pain.

1 Use heel lift to relax muscles. Apply anchor distally above malleoli and proximally at tibial tuberosity.

2 Apply medial and lateral anchor strips distal to proximal, lifting up against gravity.

3 Apply in an alternating oblique direction, forming an X over the anterior shin; work distal to proximal.

4 Apply medial and lateral anchors. Apply distal and proximal anchors.

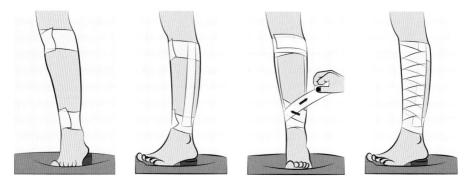

Plantar fasciitis

1 Place anchor strips around the metatarsal region of the forefoot.

2 After wrapping this area several times, use a strip to wrap from the metatarsal region near the hallux and place it around the heel before attaching at the origin behind the hallux.

3 Wrap another strip around the heel, but this time starting closer to the smaller toes. Rewrap these areas several times to add support. The area should look like an X along the midfoot region.

4 Place additional strips laterally along the wrapped area of the foot to close up gaps and reinforce the taped area.

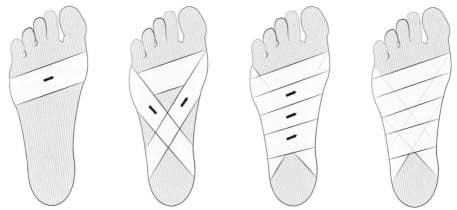

Metatarsal arch–support taping

Purpose: to provide support for the metatarsal arch.

1 Place teardrop-shaped felt pad slightly proximal to head of second to fourth metatarsals.

2 Anchor with elastic tape.

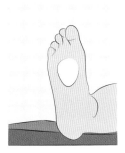 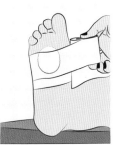 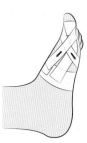

Hallux strapping

Purpose: to limit motion at the first metacarpophalangeal joint.

Protect the nail with adhesive dressing.

1 Anchor on hallux and midfoot.

2 Tape strip from distal to proximal anchor.

3 Apply additional strips until the base of the first metatarsal is covered.

4 Re-anchor.

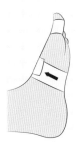 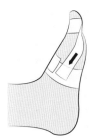 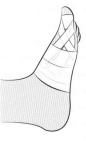

Basic kinesiology taping techniques
General ankle Ktaping

The foot is placed in flexion (toes up).

1 First strip – apply tape from the inside of the ankle underneath the heal on to the outside of the skin, at 50% stretch.

2 Second strip – follow the same direction but closer to the front of the ankle joint, at 50% stretch.

3 Third strip – apply tape around the edge of the front from inside to outside, at 50% stretch.

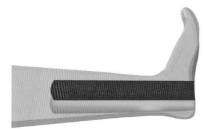 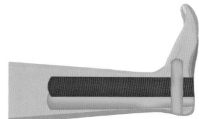

Medial ankle sprain Ktaping

Requires: 2 pieces of I-tape; a partner for taping

1 Apply one end of I-tape at the medial side of the ankle and another end to the medial side of the knee.

2 Anchor another I-tape on the inside of the ankle and apply the end of the strip as shown.

No stretch is required during application.

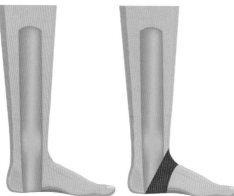

Achilles Ktaping

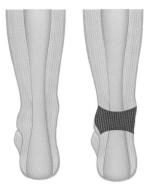 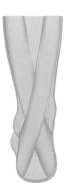

Method 1

The foot is placed into flexion (toes up). Tape is positioned from the heel to the middle of the calf with 50% stretch. An additional strip can be used along the location of the pain.

Method 2

Measure the tape. Place the centre of the tape underneath the heel bone and apply the tape. Then take one end and stretch the tape at 50%. Cross it over the Achilles tendon and attach it to the outside of the calf. Repeat with the other end, attaching the tape to the inside of the calf.

Calf Ktaping

Requires: 3 pieces of I-tape; a partner for taping

1 Place the base of I-tape at the heel and adhere the tape to the calf.

2 Place another I-tape from the lateral side of the heel to the medial side of the knee.

3 Place the last I-tape from the medial side of the heel to the lateral side of the knee.

No stretching is required during application.

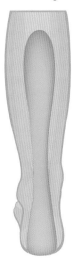 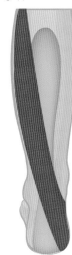 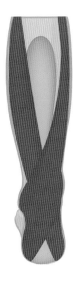

Shin splint Ktaping

Requires: 2 pieces of I-tape; self-taping is possible.

1 Place I-tape at the outside foot towards the shin while pointing the foot downwards.

2 Apply another I-tape at the inside of the foot towards the medial side of the lower leg as shown while maintaining the foot pointing downwards.

No stretch is required during application.

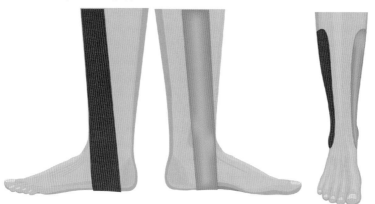

Hallux Ktaping

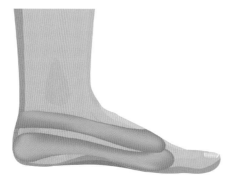

References

Bandyopadhyay, A. and Mahapatra, D. (2012) Taping in sports: A brief update. *Journal of Human Sport and Exercise* 7, 2, 544–552.

Baquie, P. (2002) Lower limb taping. *Australian Family Physician* 31, 5, 451–452.

Bassett, K.T., Lingman, S.A. and Ellis, R.F. (2010) The use and treatment efficacy of kinaesthetic taping for musculoskeletal conditions: A systematic review. *New Zealand Journal of Physiotherapy* 38, 56–62.

Best, R., Mauch, F., Böhle, C., Huth, J. and Brüggemann, P. (2014) Residual mechanical effectiveness of external ankle tape before and after competitive professional soccer performance. *Clinical Journal of Sport Medicine* 24, 1, 51–57.

Birrer, R.B. and Poole, B. (2004) Taping of sports injuries: Review of a basic skill. *Journal of Musculoskeletal Medicine 21*, 4, 197–211.

Briem, K., Eythörsdóttir, H., Magnúsdóttir, R.G., Pálmarsson, R., Rúnarsdóttir, T. and Sveinsson, T. (2011) Effects of kinesio tape compared with nonelastic sports tape and the untaped ankle during a sudden inversion perturbation in male athletes. *Journal of Orthopaedic and Sports Physical Therapy 41*, 5, 328–335.

Bunch, R.P., Bednarski, K., Holland, D. and Macinanti, R. (1985) Ankle joint support: A comparison of reusable lace-on braces with taping and wrapping. *The Physician and Sportsmedicine 13*, 5, 59–62.

Chang, H.Y., Chou, K.Y., Lin, J.J., Lin, C.F. and Wang, C.H. (2010) Immediate effect of forearm Kinesio taping on maximal grip strength and force sense in healthy collegiate athletes. *Physical Therapy in Sport 11*, 4, 122–127.

Cordova, M.L., Ingersoll, C.D. and Palmieri, R.M. (2002) Efficacy of prophylactic ankle support: An experimental perspective. *Journal of Athletic Training 37*, 4, 446–457.

Cordova, M.L., Scott, B.D., Ingersoll, C.D. and LeBlanc, M.J. (2005) Effects of ankle support on lower-extremity functional performance: A meta-analysis. *Medicine and Science in Sports and Exercise 37*, 4, 635–641.

De Ridder, R., Willems, T.M., Vanrenterghem, J. and Roosen, P. (2015) Effect of tape on dynamic postural stability in subjects with chronic ankle instability. *International Journal of Sports Medicine 36*, 4, 321–326.

Delahunt, E., McGrath, A., Doran, N. and Coughlan, G.F. (2010) Effect of taping on actual and perceived dynamic postural stability in persons with chronic ankle instability. *Archives of Physical Medicine and Rehabilitation 91*, 9, 1383–1389.

Dizon, J.M.R. and Reyes, J.J.B. (2010) A systematic review on the effectiveness of external ankle supports in the prevention of inversion ankle sprains among elite and recreational players. *Journal of Science and Medicine in Sport 13*, 3, 309–317.

Forbes, H., Thrussell, S., Haycock, N., Lohkamp, M. and White, M. (2013) The effect of prophylactic ankle support during simulated soccer activity. *Journal of Sport Rehabilitation 22*, 3, 170–176.

Grant, M.E., Steffen, K., Glasgow, P., Phillips, N., Booth, L. and Galligan, M. (2014) The role of sports physiotherapy at the London 2012 Olympic Games. *British Journal of Sports Medicine 48*, 1, 63–70.

Greene, T.A. and Hillman, S.K. (1990) Comparison of support provided by a semirigid orthosis and adhesive ankle taping before, during, and after exercise. *The American Journal of Sports Medicine 18*, 5, 498–506.

Hughes, G. and McLean, N.R. (1988) Zinc oxide tape: A useful dressing for the recalcitrant finger-tip and soft-tissue injury. *Emergency Medicine Journal 5*, 4, 223–227.

Inglés, M., Serra-Añó, P., Méndez, À.G., Zarzoso, M. *et al.* (2019) Effect of Kinesio taping and balance exercises on postural control in amateur soccer players: A randomised control trial. *Journal of Sports Sciences 37*, 24, 2853–2862.

Juchler, I., Blasimann, A., Baur, H. and Radlinger, L. (2016) The effect of Kinesio tape on neuromuscular activity of peroneus longus. *Physiotherapy Theory and Practice 32*, 2, 124–129.

Kalron, A. and Bar-Sela, S. (2013) A systematic review of the effectiveness of Kinesio taping – fact or fashion? *European Journal of Physical and Rehabilitation Medicine 49*, 5, 699–709.

Kase, K., Wallis, J. and Kase, T. (2003) *Clinical Therapeutic Applications of the Kinesio Taping Method*. Kinesio Taping Association.

Kelly, L.A., Racinais, S., Tanner, C.M., Grantham, J. and Chalabi, H. (2010) Augmented low dye taping changes muscle activation patterns and plantar pressure during treadmill running. *Journal of Orthopaedic and Sports Physical Therapy 40*, 10, 648–655.

Knight, A.C. and Weimar, W.H. (2011) Difference in response latency of the peroneus longus between the dominant and nondominant legs. *Journal of Sport Rehabilitation 20*, 3, 321–332.

Lardenoye, S., Theunissen, E., Cleffken, B., Brink, P.R., de Bie, R.A. and Poeze, M. (2012) The effect of taping versus semi-rigid bracing on patient outcome and satisfaction in ankle sprains: A prospective, randomized controlled trial. *BMC Musculoskeletal Disorders 13*, 1, 1–7.

Lim, E.C.W. and Tay, M.G.X. (2015) Kinesio taping in musculoskeletal pain and disability that lasts for more than 4 weeks: Is it time to peel off the tape and throw it out with the sweat? A systematic review with meta-analysis focused on pain and also methods of tape application. *British Journal of Sports Medicine 49*, 24, 1558–1566.

Lohrer, H., Alt, W. and Gollhofer, A. (1999) Neuromuscular properties and functional aspects of taped ankles. *The American Journal of Sports Medicine 27*, 1, 69–75.

Morris, D., Jones, D., Ryan, H. and Ryan, C.G. (2013) The clinical effects of Kinesio® Tex taping: A systematic review. *Physiotherapy Theory and Practice 29*, 4, 259–270.

Mostafavifar, M., Wertz, J. and Borchers, J. (2012) A systematic review of the effectiveness of Kinesio taping for musculoskeletal injury. *The Physician and Sportsmedicine 40*, 4, 33–40.

Nunes, G.S., Feldkircher, J.M., Tessarin, B.M., Bender, P.U., da Luz, C.M. and de Noronha, M. (2021) Kinesio taping does not improve ankle functional or performance in people with or without ankle injuries: Systematic review and meta-analysis. *Clinical Rehabilitation 35*, 2, 182–199.

Olmsted, L.C., Vela, L.I., Denegar, C.R. and Hertel, J. (2004) Prophylactic ankle taping and bracing: A numbers-needed-to-treat and cost-benefit analysis. *Journal of Athletic Training 39*, 1, 95–100.

Pamuk, U. and Yucesoy, C.A. (2015) MRI analyses show that kinesio taping affects much more than just the targeted superficial tissues and causes heterogeneous deformations within the whole limb. *Journal of Biomechanics 48*, 16, 4262–4270.

Parreira, P.D.C.S., Costa, L.D.C.M., Junior, L.C.H., Lopes, A.D. and Costa, L.O.P. (2014) Current evidence does not support the use of Kinesio taping in clinical practice: A systematic review. *Journal of Physiotherapy 60*, 1, 31–39.

Polakowski, E. (2015) *Systematic Review of Musculoskeletal Taping Methods*. Doctoral dissertation, University of Pittsburgh.

Raymond, J., Nicholson, L.L., Hiller, C.E. and Refshauge, K.M. (2012) The effect of ankle taping or bracing on proprioception in functional ankle instability: A systematic review and meta-analysis. *Journal of Science and Medicine in Sport 15*, 5, 386–392.

Riemann, B.L., Schmitz, R.J., Gale, M. and McCaw, S.T. (2002) Effect of ankle taping and bracing on vertical ground reaction forces during drop landings before and after treadmill jogging. *Journal of Orthopaedic and Sports Physical Therapy 32*, 12, 628–635.

Sawkins, K., Refshauge, K. and Kilbreath, S. (2007) The placebo effect of ankle taping in ankle instability. *Medicine and Science in Sports and Exercise 39*, 5, 781–787.

Shima, N., Maeda, A. and Hirohashi, K. (2005) Delayed latency of peroneal reflex to sudden inversion with ankle taping or bracing. *International Journal of Sports Medicine 26*, 6, 476–480.

Shin, J.C., Kim, J.H., Nam, D., Park, G.C. and Lee, J.S. (2020) Add-on effect of kinesiotape in patients with acute lateral ankle sprain: A randomized controlled trial. *Trials 21*, 1, 1–14.

Simon, J. and Donahue, M. (2013) Effect of ankle taping or bracing on creating an increased sense of confidence, stability, and reassurance when performing a dynamic-balance task. *Journal of Sport Rehabilitation 22*, 3, 229–233.

Simon, J.E. (1969) Study of the comparative effectiveness of ankle taping and ankle wrapping on the prevention of ankle injuries. *Journal of the National Athletic Trainers' Association 4*, 6–7.

Slevin, Z.M., Arnold, G.P., Wang, W. and Abboud, R.J. (2020) Immediate effect of kinesiology tape on ankle stability. *BMJ Open Sport and Exercise Medicine 6*, 1, e000604.

Stecco, C., Porzionato, A., Macchi, V., Stecco, A. *et al.* (2008) The expansions of the pectoral girdle muscles onto the brachial fascia: Morphological aspects and spatial disposition. *Cells Tissues Organs 188*, 3, 320–329.

Trégouët, P., Merland, F. and Horodyski, M.B. (2013) A comparison of the effects of ankle taping styles on biomechanics during ankle inversion. *Annals of Physical and Rehabilitation Medicine* 56, 2, 113–122.

Trofa, D.P., Obana, K.K., Herndon, C.L., Noticewala, M.S. *et al.* (2020) The evidence for common nonsurgical modalities in sports medicine, part 1: Kinesio tape, sports massage therapy, and acupuncture. *JAAOS Global Research and Reviews* 4, 1, e19.00104.

Tu, S.J., Woledge, R.C. and Morrissey, D. (2016) Does 'Kinesio tape' alter thoracolumbar fascia movement during lumbar flexion? An observational laboratory study. *Journal of Bodywork and Movement Therapies* 20, 4, 898–905.

Wang, Y., Gu, Y., Chen, J., Luo, W. *et al.* (2018) Kinesio taping is superior to other taping methods in ankle functional performance improvement: A systematic review and meta-analysis. *Clinical Rehabilitation* 32, 11, 1472–1481.

Wilkerson, G.B. (2002) Biomechanical and neuromuscular effects of ankle taping and bracing. *Journal of Athletic Training* 37, 4, 436–445.

Williams, S., Whatman, C., Hume, P.A. and Sheerin, K. (2012) Kinesio taping in treatment and prevention of sports injuries: A meta-analysis of the evidence for its effectiveness. *Sports Medicine* 42, 2, 153–164.

Wilson, B. and Bialocerkowski, A. (2015) The effects of Kinesiotape applied to the lateral aspect of the ankle: Relevance to ankle sprains – a systematic review. *PLOS ONE* 10, 6, e0124214.

Yin, L. and Wang, L. (2020) Acute effect of kinesiology taping on postural stability in individuals with unilateral chronic ankle instability. *Frontiers in Physiology* 2000, 11, 192.

Yoon, J.Y., An, D.H. and Oh, J.S. (2013) Plantarflexor and dorsiflexor activation during inclined walking with and without modified mobilization with movement using tape in women with limited ankle dorsiflexion. *Journal of Physical Therapy Science* 25, 8, 993–995.

Zwiers, R., Vuurberg, G., Blankevoort, L. and Kerkhoffs, G.M.M.J. (2016) Taping and bracing in the prevention of ankle sprains: Current concepts. *Journal of ISAKOS* 1, 6, 304–310.

Chapter 14

Exercise Rehabilitation for the Foot and Ankle

IAIN BARROWMAN

Within the worlds of health and fitness and physical medicine, the terms 'physical activity', 'physical fitness' and 'exercise' are very similar constructs. In common usage, these terms are sometimes used interchangeably. However, they all pertain to different concepts and have their own distinct definitions (Garber *et al.*, 2011). The World Health Organization (2020) refers to 'physical activity' as any bodily movement resulting from skeletal muscle contraction that elevates energy expenditure above resting levels. In contrast, physical fitness is the body's ability to carry out work-related, sports or daily activities with ample strength, energy and vigour. In other words, it refers to an optimal state of health in which the body can function efficiently and effectively without getting easily fatigued (Caspersen *et al.*, 1985).

Exercise, on the other hand, is often recognised as a subcategory of physical activity. It is usually defined as an activity that requires repetitive physical effort and is planned and structured with the aim to sustain or improve health and fitness (Garber *et al.*, 2011; Wasfy and Baggish, 2016). Exercise can also be carried out for a specific purpose such as rehabilitation after an illness or injury. It offers many benefits to patients including reduced inflammation, decreased anxiety, lessened fatigue, faster recovery and improved mood and sleep. All of these are necessary for good general health, along with the repair and regeneration of soft-tissue structures.

This chapter discusses what exercise rehabilitation is, how to structure a rehabilitation programme and the clinical relevance of exercise therapy for foot and ankle injuries.

What is exercise rehabilitation?

Exercise rehabilitation, exercise therapy or therapeutic exercise is one of the most powerful and beneficial manual therapy modalities that manual therapists have at their disposal. Exercise therapy is a set of proven physical activities designed and planned to achieve specific treatment goals. It can be prescribed for the prevention, management and rehabilitation of a variety of chronic musculoskeletal, cardiorespiratory and neurological pathologies (Smidt *et al.*, 2005). In fact, the therapy involves a series of physical activities designed to restore function, correct impairments and improve the patient's overall health and well-being (American Physical Therapy Association, 2001).

In clinical studies, exercise therapy has been shown to be a safe and effective solution for managing a range of chronic conditions that do not require potentially harmful and costly prescription medications, steroidal injections or invasive surgery (Skou *et al.*, 2018). The available evidence supports the use of exercise therapy in the treatment of no less than 26 chronic conditions. In fact, the current evidence suggests that the effects of exercise therapy are comparable to those of conventional medical treatment in selected cases. In addition, in special situations, exercise may outperform the conservative treatments or add to their effect (Pedersen and Saltin, 2015). On the other hand, there is currently no evidence to suggest that exercise therapy is harmful. However, a possible reason for this could be the poor reporting of adverse effects in clinical studies, particularly randomised controlled trials (Lin *et al.*, 2020).

General guidelines for exercise rehabilitation

Exercise therapy should be tailored to every single patient, centred on their case and dictated by their goals. The end goal of rehabilitation through exercise should be returning the patient to their full fitness, ideally at better or similar levels before the injury, surgery or illness. The duration, length, intensity and complexity of the exercises can vary depending on the age, condition, goals and resources available to the patient. Therefore, manual therapists should proceed with an individualised approach and have a clear idea about which forms of exercise are more suitable for an individual patient. They should also be able to adapt the exercise prescription if the patient does not respond positively (American College of Sports Medicine, 2006; Wade, 2009).

The therapist should ensure that the patient is educated on the exercise rehabilitation programme, what its goals are and why certain exercises have been selected. This will help to foster a therapeutic alliance. To enhance self-efficacy, the therapist may also focus on the personal preferences of the patient such as swimming and walking, or training in a less busy environment or with the therapist present. Doing so, the therapist can make the exercise sessions more enjoyable for the patient, along with promoting positive behavioural changes (Garber *et al.*, 2011).

How to structure an exercise rehabilitation programme

Rehabilitation specialists generally develop an exercise prescription after a full assessment of the patient's condition. The acronym FITT (frequency, intensity, time and type) is commonly utilised to characterise the exercise prescription. The American College of Sports Medicine (ACSM) has recently modified this acronym by adding two new components (i.e. volume of exercise and progression of physical activity) (Pescatello *et al.*, 2013). With this addition, they produced the new acronym FITT-VP (see Table 14.1).

Table 14.1 ACSM recommended fundamental components of exercise

Frequency	The number of times an exercise session needs to be carried out (typically per week or per day).
Intensity	The intensity at which the individual will train. This can be measured by tools such as the BORG scale, heart rate or percentage of one rep max.
Time	The duration of the session.
Type	The type(s) of skill and health-related components that are focused on during the session.
Volume	A measurement of the number of exercises, and their number of sets and repetitions.
Progression	The progressions of exercises that can be selected as the individual progresses through the programme. This is an essential component that ensures a linear progression.

Dosage

The term 'dosage' is frequently used in the exercise rehabilitation literature. In the context of exercise therapy, this term usually refers to the number of sessions per week, the volume of exercises each day or the sum of repetitions to be performed (Swain, 2013). No consensus, however, currently exists among researchers regarding the parameters (e.g. frequency and duration of exercise, the volume of sets and reps) of an exercise therapy protocol for a given condition (Young *et al.*, 2018). Nevertheless, this does not mean that exercise prescriptions do not follow evidence-based principles.

It is of critical importance to personalise the exercise intensity based on the overall condition and unique needs of each patient. Luan *et al.* (2019) suggested utilising several measures to determine the exercise intensity, including oxygen uptake level, heart rate reserve, target heart rate and perceived exertion rate. In minor to moderate levels of the disease, the therapist can adopt a moderate-intensity exercise protocol for the patient. If the overall condition of the patient seems satisfactory, high-intensity training can also be adopted. However, in severe, late-stage, post-surgery cases, the therapist should go with a low-intensity training protocol and increase the load intensity gradually (Swain, 2013).

Manual therapists should also make sure that the exercise prescription is relatable to the varying components of the physical health domain, including health-related, medical-related and skill-related components. This is important because a majority of people live a more sedentary lifestyle and are not used to being physically active to a moderate or high degree (Pescatello *et al.*, 2013). On the other hand, physical inactivity has been a leading risk factor for a number of chronic diseases such as dementia, osteoarthritis, heart disease, diabetes and cancer (Booth *et al.*, 2012). Hence, the exercise programme has historically been focused on skill-related and health-related components.

However, given the varying nature of musculoskeletal conditions, manual therapists should also allow for the medical-related components in their exercise rehabilitation programme. They must fully understand the limitations and contraindications to exercise for specific patient populations. This is especially important for patients who are suffering from respiratory conditions such as asthma or emphysema, or cardiovascular conditions such as angina or myocarditis. In addition, manual therapists should also bear in mind that they need to support the patient at various stages of the rehabilitation and healing timeframe. Hence, they must prescribe and design a bespoke exercise rehabilitation programme that addresses various risk factors including age, any pre-existing medical condition(s), training age and outcome desire (Bovend'Eerdt *et al.*, 2009; Wade, 2009; Wasfy and Baggish, 2016; Dubois and Esculier, 2020).

Table 14.2 Examples of individual components of the physical health domain

Health-related fitness components	Skill-related fitness components	Medical-related fitness components
Cardiovascular endurance	Speed	Musculoskeletal
Muscular endurance	Power	Cardiovascular

Muscular strength	Agility	Lymphatic
Flexibility	Balance	Neurologic
Body composition	Coordination	Respiratory
	Reaction time	Digestive and urogenital
		Integumentary
		Endocrine and immunity

Adapted from American College of Sports Medicine (2006)

Considerations for foot and ankle exercise rehabilitation

Ankle or foot injuries can happen to individuals of any age and are not specific to active people. A recent population-based study by Ferguson *et al.* (2019) reported that about 3% of the UK population of all ages are affected by foot and ankle conditions. The study also reported around 34,000 referrals to physiotherapists during the four-year period between 2010 and 2013. These estimates, however, are found to be much higher for the older population (≥ 45 years). Of the various musculoskeletal injuries, ankle sprains of varying degrees are one of the most common of all injuries. Ankle sprains account for nearly 5% of all casualty room visits in the UK per annum, which means approximately 5600 incidences of ankle sprains occur per day (Bestwick-Stevenson *et al.*, 2021).

Achilles tendinopathy is another common overuse injury of the foot and ankle complex (Abat *et al.*, 2018). The injury is often seen due to repeated overuse or trauma to the Achilles tendon. In the UK, it is estimated to affect over 150,000 people annually (Kearney *et al.*, 2013). In a recent study, however, O'Neill *et al.* (2017) suggested that the prevalence of Achilles tendinopathy in the general population is about 2%. In more severe cases, an Achilles tendon rupture (ATR) can occur, which accounts for roughly 4500 cases per annum in the UK (Boyd *et al.*, 2015). ATR is usually caused by overstretching of the tendon beyond its capacity (Shamrock and Varacallo, 2021). The injury is generally seen in active populations, mostly occurring during participation in sports either through an acute injury or by way of tendinopathies from a chronic background (Klatte-Schulz *et al.*, 2018). However, this injury can also happen to anyone with no past background or history of involvement in active sports.

Achilles tendinopathy

Achilles tendinopathy is also known as Achilles tendinitis, tendinosis, tenosynovitis or paratenonitis (Almekinders and Temple, 1998; Yu *et al.*, 2013; Klatte-Schulz *et al.*, 2018). The suffix 'osis' is indicative of a degenerative process, while 'itis' refers to an inflammatory disorder. Maffulli *et al.* (1998) suggested that the correct terminology for this condition should be tendinopathy due to its histopathology and clinical signs. This is because it is not always clear whether the condition is purely degenerative or inflammatory in nature; therefore, the terminology of tendinopathy is more appropriate.

There are two classifications of Achilles tendinopathy, which relate to the condition's anatomical location. The first is insertional (at the calcaneus tendon junction) and the second is non-insertional (2–3 inches from the proximal insertion on to the calcaneus) (Almekinders and Temple, 1998).

The management for Achilles tendinopathy can vary between practitioners, with some advocating rest for a period while following the PRICE protocol (protect, rest, ice, compression, elevation), and others advocating to maintain activity levels, with the patient exercising through tolerable discomfort (up to but not into pain). In an acute setting with a new onset of pain, rest is initially advisable, and high-intensity activities should be stopped completely. However, prolonged inactivity may worsen the condition. If the condition is chronic and/or repetitive in nature, then the patient would most probably benefit from education on activity modification along with a robust exercise rehabilitation programme while still partaking in their chosen discipline or activity (Klatte-Schulz *et al.*, 2018).

Exercise rehabilitation is currently the best-researched intervention for Achilles tendinopathy with the highest volume of clinical evidence (Yu *et al.*, 2013; University of British Columbia, 2021). The patient should start a phased tendon-loading programme with gentle exercise and gradually increase the intensity. This should be started after the initial assessment and last around two weeks.

A great resource for the management of Achilles tendinopathy is the Achilles Tendinopathy Toolkit (University of British Columbia, 2021), which is an evidence-based clinical decision-making tool designed to provide clinicians with clear knowledge and advice on the best management of the condition. The toolkit includes a list of interventions with a summary of the strength of evidence, key messages and recommendations for practice for an array of interventions used by physiotherapists.

Achilles tendon rupture

There is currently no consensus as to how best to manage or treat ATR. Treatment options range from minimally invasive surgical options to more conventional open surgeries. Rehabilitation is a key aspect following Achilles tendon repair surgery, which usually aims for an early return to pre-injury levels of activity. Rehabilitation has also been reported to be effective in ATR patients treated with non-invasive management. In fact, Wu *et al.* (2016) recently demonstrated functional rehabilitation methods to be as effective as the surgical route. However, a cautious approach needs to be taken so that no further tendon rupture or elongation happens (Brumann *et al.*, 2014).

On the other hand, there is still a great debate regarding whether a more functional approach to the rehabilitation programme is more effective than a traditional approach (Zhao *et al.*, 2017). Although the evidence in support of early weight-bearing is now increasing, no consensus has yet been reached on the preferred rehabilitation protocol. Regardless of the debate, manual therapists should carefully consider several factors before selecting any interventions for the treatment of a patient's injury. These include the patient's age, activity levels, mental readiness to return to activity/sport and pre-existing comorbidities (Shamrock and Varacallo, 2021).

Timeline for accelerated functional approach

The timeframes in the protocol are approximate. Not every patient with an ATR will follow the same timeline. Progression should be based upon the clinical presentation as well as continued assessment. A consistent definition of what constitutes early functional rehabilitation has not been established (Brumann *et al.*, 2014; Zellers *et al.*, 2019). Some of the principles within this method are:

- plantar flexor strengthening
- gait education
- foot strengthening
- balance and proprioception development.

Weeks 0–2: The patient should be instructed to avoid dorsiflexion or plantarflexion, with the foot and ankle ideally being immobilised in an air cast with a wedge to hold the ankle in approximately 30° plantarflexion. There should be minimal weight-bearing on the affected side, and crutches should be used for ambulation.

Weeks 2–6: The patient should be instructed to begin plantarflexion and dorsiflexion exercises, along with inversion and eversion. The patient should continue to use crutches to support weight-bearing.

Weeks 6–8: The wedge in the air cast should be reduced to allow the ankle to reach a neutral position. During this stage, some light stretching of the dorsiflexors may be used, along with hydrotherapy if available. Resistance exercises may also be introduced at this stage.

Weeks 8–12: The patient should be weaned from the boot and continue to progress with exercises focusing on strength, flexibility and proprioception.

Weeks > 12: This stage will see the patient further work on strength, flexibility and proprioception of the foot and ankle, seeking to return to pre-injury levels. Patients should be encouraged to work on dynamic and plyometric exercises and sport-specific exercises aiming to improve on pre-injury levels of strength, balance, proprioception and flexibility.

Timeline for a traditional approach

The traditional method includes 6–8 weeks of non-weight-bearing with cast immobilisation, followed by several weeks in a boot. This is to ensure that the tendon is completely healed in the proper position. The initial goal following the removal of the air cast/boot should be to improve the range of motion of the ankle. Once the ankle is able to move in all planes without much discomfort, the therapist should focus on strengthening the muscles of the lower leg. This should incorporate the muscles on the anterior and lateral aspect of the lower leg as well (Zhao *et al.*, 2017; Shamrock and Varacallo, 2021).

Weeks 0–8: During this period, the patient's ankle should be fixed in place, and ambulation should be assisted with crutches. However, during this time the rehabilitation of the patient can begin with a focus on developing trunk strength, joint mobility and tissue flexibility on the contralateral leg as well as the knee and hip joint of the affected leg.

Weeks 8–12: Once the cast is removed, the ankle should be passively mobilised along with the joints in the foot. Exercises focusing on retraining of gait, low-level strengthening and proprioceptive work can now begin.

Weeks 12–24: The patient should start doing more dynamic movements such as walking on the toes, lunging, walking and jogging. A focus should still be on developing the basics of strength, balance, proprioception and flexibility.

Weeks > 24: During this stage, the patient may be able to begin a run programme, under the supervision of the surgeon or manual therapist, if the patient meets the desired outcome measures.

Ankle sprain

The available evidence from the peer-reviewed literature suggests that the treatment of choice for ankle sprains should be progressive weight-bearing with functional ankle support, particularly for grade I and II sprains (level 2 evidence). Rigid immobilisation for a short duration (< 10 days) has also been found to be helpful in the treatment of ankle sprains, especially for grade III injuries (level 2 evidence) (Halabchi and Hassabi, 2020; Tran and McCormack, 2020).

In practice, the RICE (rest, ice, compression, elevation) and ICE (ice, compression, elevation) protocols have historically been utilised in the first few days following an ankle sprain. However, the current evidence does not recommend the use of RICE nor ICE, as neither outlines a proper guideline for the management and rehabilitation of subacute and chronic stages of tissue healing (Block, 2010; Bleakley *et al.*, 2012a, 2012b; Van den Bekerom *et al.*, 2012). Several other non-pharmacological modalities have also been found ineffective in the management of ankle sprains (level 3 evidence). These include prolotherapy, ultrasound therapy, acupuncture, low-level lasers, electrotherapy, whole-body vibration, shortwave diathermy and Bioptron light therapy (Tran and McCormack, 2020).

The mainstay for the treatment of acute ankle sprain is early mobilisation through exercise therapy. This has been supported by a growing body of evidence (Halabchi and Hassabi, 2020). In fact, exercise-based rehabilitation has been shown to significantly reduce the recurrence of sprains and functional instability of the ankle compared with the standard programme alone (Bleakley *et al.*, 2019; Wagemans *et al.*, 2022). Exercise therapy programmes can be supervised or home-based. However, there is controversy regarding whether supervised rehabilitation is more beneficial than the usual care alone in terms of recovery.

To date, various types of exercises have been suggested for the rehabilitation of ankle sprains. As stated above, however, these programmes need to be progressive and comprehensive. Nevertheless, it should be noted that no consensus has yet been reached on the optimal exercise content and parameters for the management of ankle sprain (Wagemans *et al.*, 2022). Below are some of the exercises recommended in the peer-reviewed literature:

- range-of-motion exercises

- stretching and strengthening exercises

- proprioceptive exercises

- balance or water-based exercises

- sport-specific functional exercises.

On the other hand, the efficacy of exercise therapy can also be amplified by combining it with manual therapy (level 3 evidence). In fact, in patients with an acute lateral ankle sprain, the clinical guideline presented by Vuurberg *et al.* (2018) recommends the inclusion of manual mobilisation in exercise rehabilitation programmes to increase ankle range of motion and enhance functional recovery.

Manual mobilisation of the ankle joint usually involves active dorsiflexion and anteroposterior talus mobilisation, which may be carried out in both weight-bearing and non-weight-bearing positions. Other methods commonly applied by manual therapists include lymphatic drainage massage, soft-tissue mobilisation and talocrural distraction manipulation.

General management (sets, reps, training volume and type of exercises)

There is a lack of adequate data in the current literature on the optimal exercise type, content and parameters for the best management of foot and ankle injuries. This has also been demonstrated in recent meta-analyses on acute ankle sprain rehabilitation. After pooling data from 14 randomised controlled trials, Wagemans *et al.* (2022) found that rehabilitation time per session varied considerably across studies, ranging from 10 to 60 minutes, although 30 minutes per session was reported to be a standard approach. In addition, total rehabilitation time also varied greatly, ranging from 3.5 to 21 hours. On the other hand, Bleakley *et al.* (2019) found a greater emphasis on the postural balance exercises in the management of acute ankle sprains, followed by strength, agility and power-based exercises.

Young *et al.* (2018) conducted a systematic review to determine the optimal doses of exercise therapy associated with greater treatment effect sizes in individuals with common musculoskeletal disorders of the foot and ankle. The authors found that three sets of 15 repetitions two times per day seven days a week was a common dose for eccentric exercises aimed at treating Achilles tendinopathy. Beyer *et al.* (2015) utilised the same prescription in a home-based exercise programme and reported positive effects in relation to pain reduction and functional recovery. However, using the same prescription three times per week, Yu *et al.* (2013) found no significant therapeutic effects in support of sets or reps.

Disclaimer

- The timelines and prescriptions discussed herein are for guidance only.

- The suggestions for specific training modes are primarily provided to make this review of practical use. They were mainly included based on the current evidence from the available literature and clinical practice experience of the authors.

References

Abat, F., Alfredson, H., Cucchiarini, M., Madry, H. *et al.* (2018) Current trends in tendinopathy: Consensus of the ESSKA basic science committee. Part II: treatment options. *Journal of Experimental Orthopaedics* 5, 1, 38.

Almekinders, L.C. and Temple, J.D. (1998) Etiology, diagnosis, and treatment of tendonitis: An analysis of the literature. *Medicine and Science in Sports and Exercise* 30, 8, 1183–1190.

American College of Sports Medicine (2006) *General Principles of Exercise Prescription.* ACSM's guidelines for exercise testing and prescription, www.acsm.org/docs/default-source/publications-files/acsms-exercise-testing-prescription.pdf?sfvrsn=111e9306_4

American Physical Therapy Association (2001) Guide to Physical Therapist Practice. Second Edition. *Physical Therapy* 81, 1, 9–746.

Bestwick-Stevenson, T., Wyatt, L.A., Palmer, D., Ching, A. *et al.* (2021) Incidence and risk factors for poor ankle functional recovery, and the development and progression of posttraumatic ankle osteoarthritis after significant ankle ligament injury (SALI): The SALI cohort study protocol. *BMC Musculoskeletal Disorders* 22, 1, 1–11.

Beyer, R., Kongsgaard, M., Hougs Kjær, B., Øhlenschlæger, T., Kjær, M. and Magnusson, S.P. (2015) Heavy slow resistance versus eccentric training as treatment for Achilles tendinopathy: A randomized controlled trial. *The American Journal of Sports Medicine* 43, 1704–1711.

Bleakley, C.M., Glasgow, P. and MacAuley, D.C. (2012a) PRICE needs updating, should we call the POLICE? *British Journal of Sports Medicine* 46, 4, 220–221.

Bleakley, C.M., Glasgow, P. and Webb, M.J. (2012b) Cooling an acute muscle injury: Can basic scientific theory translate into the clinical setting? *British Journal of Sports Medicine 46*, 4, 296–298.

Bleakley, C.M., Taylor, J.B., Dischiavi, S.L., Doherty, C. and Delahunt, E. (2019) Rehabilitation exercises reduce reinjury post ankle sprain, but the content and parameters of an optimal exercise program have yet to be established: A systematic review and meta-analysis. *Archives of Physical Medicine and Rehabilitation 100*, 7, 1367–1375.

Block, J.E. (2010) Cold and compression in the management of musculoskeletal injuries and orthopedic operative procedures: A narrative review. *Open Access Journal of Sports Medicine 1*, 105–113.

Booth, F.W., Roberts, C.K. and Laye, M.J. (2012) Lack of exercise is a major cause of chronic diseases. *Comprehensive Physiology 2*, 2, 1143–1211.

Bovend'Eerdt, T.J.H., Botell, R.E. and Wade, D.T. (2009) Writing SMART rehabilitation goals and achieving goal attainment scaling: A practical guide. *Clinical Rehabilitation 23*, 4, 352–361.

Boyd, R.P., Dimock, R., Solan, M.C. and Porter, E. (2015) Achilles tendon rupture: How to avoid missing the diagnosis. *British Journal of General Practice 65*, 641, 668–669.

Brumann, M., Baumbach, S.F., Mutschler, W. and Polzer, H. (2014) Accelerated rehabilitation following Achilles tendon repair after acute rupture – development of an evidence-based treatment protocol. *Injury 45*, 11, 1782–1790.

Burke, S.M., Shapcott, K.M., Carron, A.V. and Eys, M.A. (2008) A Qualitative Examination of the Reasons for University- and Middle-Aged Women's Preferences for Strength Training Contexts. In L.T. Allerton and G.P. Rutherfode (eds) *Exercise and Women's Health: New Research*. Nova Science Publishers.

Caspersen, C.J., Powell, K.E. and Christenson, G. (1985) Physical activity, exercise, and physical fitness: Definitions and distinctions for health-related research. *Public Health Reports 100*, 2, 126–131.

Dubois, B. and Esculier, J. (2020) Soft-tissue injuries simply need PEACE and LOVE. *British Journal of Sports Medicine 54*, 2, 72–73.

Ferguson, R., Culliford, D., Prieto-Alhambra, D., Pinedo-Villanueva, R. *et al.* (2019) Encounters for foot and ankle pain in UK primary care: A population-based cohort study of CPRD data. *British Journal of General Practice 69*, 683, e422–e429.

Garber, C.E., Blissmer, B., Deschenes, M.R., Franklin, B.A. *et al.* (2011) American College of Sports Medicine position stand. Quantity and quality of exercise for developing and maintaining cardiorespiratory, musculoskeletal, and neuromotor fitness in apparently healthy adults: Guidance for prescribing exercise. *Medicine and Science in Sports and Exercise 43*, 7, 1334–1359.

Halabchi, F. and Hassabi, M. (2020) Acute ankle sprain in athletes: Clinical aspects and algorithmic approach. *World Journal of Orthopedics 11*, 12, 534–558.

Kearney, R.S., Parsons, N. and Costa, M.L. (2013) Achilles tendinopathy management: A pilot randomised controlled trial comparing platelet-rich plasma injection with an eccentric loading programme. *Bone and Joint Research 2*, 10, 227–232.

Klatte-Schulz, F., Minkwitz, S., Schmock, A., Bormann, N. *et al.* (2018) Different Achilles tendon pathologies show distinct histological and molecular characteristics. *International Journal of Molecular Sciences 19*, 2, 404.

Lin, I., Wiles, L., Waller, R., Goucke, R. *et al.* (2020) What does best practice care for musculoskeletal pain look like? Eleven consistent recommendations from high-quality clinical practice guidelines: Systematic review. *British Journal of Sports Medicine 54*, 2, 79–86.

Luan, X., Tian, X., Zhang, H., Huang, R. *et al.* (2019) Exercise as a prescription for patients with various diseases. *Journal of Sport and Health Science 8*, 5, 422–441.

Maffulli, N., Khan, K.M. and Puddu, G. (1998) Overuse tendon conditions: Time to change a confusing terminology. *Arthroscopy: The Journal of Arthroscopic and Related Surgery 14*, 8, 840–843.

O'Neill, S., Barry, S. and Watson, P. (2017) O9: The epidemiology of Achilles tendinopathy in UK runners. *Online Journal of Rural Nursing and Health Care* 17, 1, S11.

Pedersen, B.K. and Saltin, B. (2015) Exercise as medicine – evidence for prescribing exercise as therapy in 26 different chronic diseases. *Scandinavian Journal of Medicine and Science in Sports* 25, 1–72.

Pescatello, L.S., Arena, R., Riebe, D. and Thompson, P.D. (2013) Sneak peek: Preview of ACSM's Guidelines for Exercise Testing and Prescription, ninth edition. *ACSM's Health and Fitness Journal* 17, 2, 16–20.

Shamrock, A.G. and Varacallo, M. (2021) Achilles Tendon Rupture. StatPearls [Internet], www.ncbi.nlm.nih.gov/books/NBK430844

Skou, S.T., Pedersen, B.K., Abbott, J.H., Patterson, B. and Barton, C. (2018) Physical activity and exercise therapy benefit more than just symptoms and impairments in people with hip and knee osteoarthritis. *The Journal of Orthopaedic and Sports Physical Therapy* 48, 6, 439–447.

Smidt, N., De Vet, H.C.W., Bouter, L.M., Dekker, J. *et al.* (2005) Effectiveness of exercise therapy: A best-evidence summary of systematic reviews. *Australian Journal of Physiotherapy* 51, 2, 71–85.

Swain, D.P. (2013) *ACSM's Resource Manual for Guidelines for Exercise Testing and Prescription*, 7th edn. Wolters Kluwer Health/Lippincott Williams & Wilkins.

Tran, K. and McCormack, S. (2020) *Exercise for the Treatment of Ankle Sprain: A Review of Clinical Effectiveness and Guidelines.* Canadian Agency for Drugs and Technologies in Health, www.ncbi.nlm.nih.gov/books/NBK563007

University of British Columbia (2021) Achilles Tendinopathy Toolkit. University of British Columbia, https://physicaltherapy.med.ubc.ca/physical-therapy-knowledge-broker/tendinopathy-toolkit

Van den Bekerom, M.P.J., Struijs, P.A.A., Blankevoort, L., Welling, L., Van Dijk, C.N. and Kerkhoffs, G.M.M. (2012) What is the evidence for rest, ice, compression, and elevation therapy in the treatment of ankle sprains in adults? *Journal of Athletic Training* 47, 4, 435–443.

Vuurberg, G., Hoorntje, A., Wink, L.M., Van Der Doelen, B.F. *et al.* (2018) Diagnosis, treatment and prevention of ankle sprains: Update of an evidence-based clinical guideline. *British Journal of Sports Medicine* 52, 15, 956–956.

Wade, D.T. (2009) Goal setting in rehabilitation: An overview of what, why and how. *Clinical Rehabilitation* 23, 4, 291–295.

Wagemans, J., Bleakley, C., Taeymans, J., Schurz, A.P. *et al.* (2022) Exercise-based rehabilitation reduces reinjury following acute lateral ankle sprain: A systematic review update with meta-analysis. *PLOS ONE* 17, 2, e0262023.

Wasfy, M.M. and Baggish, A.L. (2016) Exercise dose in clinical practice. *Circulation* 133, 23, 2297–2313.

World Health Organization (2020) Physical activity: What is physical activity? www.who.int/news-room/fact-sheets/detail/physical-activity

Wu, Y., Lin, L., Li, H., Zhao, Y. *et al.* (2016) Is surgical intervention more effective than non-surgical treatment for acute Achilles tendon rupture? A systematic review of overlapping meta-analyses. *International Journal of Surgery* 36, Pt A, 305–311.

Young, J.L., Rhon, D.I., De Zoete, R.M.J., Cleland, J.A. and Snodgrass, S.J. (2018) The influence of dosing on effect size of exercise therapy for musculoskeletal foot and ankle disorders: A systematic review. *Revista Brasileira De Fisioterapia* 22, 1, 20–32.

Yu, J., Park, D. and Lee, G. (2013) Effect of eccentric strengthening on pain, muscle strength, endurance, and functional fitness factors in male patients with Achilles tendinopathy. *American Journal of Physical Medicine and Rehabilitation* 92, 1, 68–76.

Zellers, J.A., Christensen, M., Kjaer, I.L., Rathleff, M.S. and Silbernagel, K.G. (2019) Defining components of early functional rehabilitation for acute Achilles tendon rupture: A systematic review. *Orthopaedic Journal of Sports Medicine* 7, 11, 2325967119884071.

Zhao, J.G., Meng, X.H., Liu, L., Zeng, X.T. and Kan, S.L. (2017) Early functional rehabilitation versus traditional immobilization for surgical Achilles tendon repair after acute rupture: A systematic review of overlapping meta-analyses. *Scientific Reports* 7, 39871.

Exercise Rehabilitation for the Foot and Ankle

Fundamental Strength

Plantarflexion, dorsiflexion, inversion and eversion banded exercises

Level 2 Progressive Strength

Single-leg heel raise, step up and down, elevated heel touches – low-level, seated dorsiflexion, split squat

Level 3 Progressive Strength

Single-leg heel raise – deficit, seated double-leg heel raise – increased weight, elevated heel touches – increased height, FFE split squat, standing dorsiflexion

Level 4 Progressive Strength

Single-leg heel raise – weighted (with/without deficit), seated double-leg heel raise – increased weight, elevated heel touches – increased height, FFE split squat (with weight), standing dorsiflexion

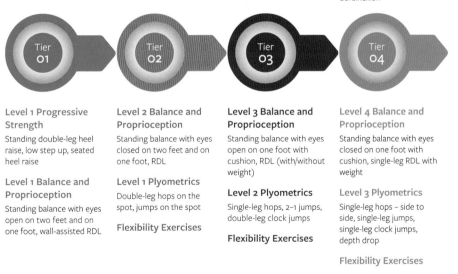

Level 1 Progressive Strength

Standing double-leg heel raise, low step up, seated heel raise

Level 1 Balance and Proprioception

Standing balance with eyes open on two feet and on one foot, wall-assisted RDL

Level 2 Balance and Proprioception

Standing balance with eyes closed on two feet and on one foot, RDL

Level 1 Plyometrics

Double-leg hops on the spot, jumps on the spot

Flexibility Exercises

Level 3 Balance and Proprioception

Standing balance with eyes open on one foot with cushion, RDL (with/without weight)

Level 2 Plyometrics

Single-leg hops, 2–1 jumps, double-leg clock jumps

Flexibility Exercises

Level 4 Balance and Proprioception

Standing balance with eyes closed on one foot with cushion, single-leg RDL with weight

Level 3 Plyometrics

Single-leg hops – side to side, single-leg jumps, single-leg clock jumps, depth drop

Flexibility Exercises

Ankle rehabilitation flowchart
FFE = front foot elevated; RDL = Romanian deadlift

Strength development

Here we have broken it down into two sections: fundamental strength and progressive strength. Although there are no hard definitions, the former is primarily used to treat foot and ankle issues at the baseline level – for example, on first loading the lower limb after the removal of a cast post-surgery.

However, in some circumstances the use of these exercises may be detrimental and may deload the patient's tissues, which will not cause the required level of stimulus to see positive adaptations. For example, a patient with chronic ankle instability may not benefit from these fundamental exercises as the loads that they are exerting and managing through carrying out activities of daily living is already much greater than that of a resistance band. These patients will receive much greater benefit from the former set of exercises.

Balance and proprioception

Balance is the maintenance of a position without moving for a given period (Haff and Triplett, 2016). In manual therapy, balance may sometimes be referred to as postural control or stability, or even equilibrium.

Within balance itself, there are two types:

- **static:** the ability to remain static in a fixed posture (Bressel *et al.*, 2007)

- **dynamic:** the ability to remain stable while performing a movement or series of movements which require a stable base of support (Winter *et al.*, 1990).

Proprioception is an afferent response to the stimulation of mechanoreceptors, Golgi tendon organs, skin, muscle, ligaments and tendons. It helps to control balance, posture and the person's sense of their body's position in space and time (Häkkinen, 1985).

The receptors responsible for this are called proprioceptors, which are small specialised sensory receptors that are responsible for relaying information to the CNS on the body's position in space and time, enabling us to carry out coordinated movements and the maintenance of muscle tone. Two of the most important proprioceptors are the Golgi tendon organs and the muscle spindles.

Plyometrics

Exercises which fall under the bracket of plyometrics are designed to enable the muscle to reach its maximal force output in the shortest possible time. They will at some stage become an integral part of the programme (Wilt, 1975).

The true definition of a plyometric exercise is one that loads the musculo-tendinous junction quickly, while minimising ground contact time. Exercises that would fit this definition are depth drop variations and hurdle jump variations (Davies *et al.*, 2015).

Flexibility

Flexibility is a measure of the available range of motion at a joint or a series of joints. Like balance, it can be broken down into two types or components:

- **static:** the range of movement at a joint and its surrounding tissues during a passive movement or stretch (Haff and Triplett, 2016)

- **dynamic:** the range of motion during active movements, which requires muscular contractions (Haff and Triplett, 2016).

There are four main types of stretch:

- **static:** a slow constant stretch held for several seconds or minutes (Bandy *et al.*, 1994)

- **ballistic:** typically a movement which is not held but rather 'bounced' in, which requires muscular contraction.

- **dynamic:** also known as a mobility drill – this may be carried out in a sports-specific setting such as walking hurdle drills (Mann and Jones, 1999)

- **proprioceptive neuromuscular facilitation:** usually requiring a partner, performed using concentric and isometric actions (Sady *et al.*, 1982).

References

Bandy, W.D., Irion, J.M. and Walker, J.M. (1994) The effect of time on static stretch on the flexibility of the hamstring muscles. *Physical Therapy* 74, 9, 845–852.

Bressel, E., Yonker, J.C., Kras, J. and Heath, E.M. (2007) Comparison of static and dynamic balance in female collegiate soccer, basketball, and gymnastics athletes. *Journal of Athletic Training 42*, 1, 42–46.

Davies, G., Riemann, B.L. and Manske, R. (2015) Current concepts of plyometric exercise. *International Journal of Sports Physical Therapy 10*, 6, 760–786.

Haff, G. and Triplett, N.T. (2016) *Essentials of Strength Training and Conditioning*. Human Kinetics.

Häkkinen, K. (1985) Factors influencing trainability of muscular strength during short term and prolonged training. *National Strength and Conditioning Association Journal 7*, 2, 32–37.

Mann, D.P. and Jones, M.T. (1999) Guidelines to the implementation of a dynamic stretching program. *Strength and Conditioning 21*, 6, 53–55.

Sady, S.P., Wortman, M. and Blanke, D. (1982) Flexibility training: Ballistic, static or proprioceptive neuromuscular facilitation? *Archives of Physical Medicine and Rehabilitation 63*, 6, 261–263.

Wilt, F. (1975) Plyometrics: What it is and how it works. *Athletic Journal 55*, 5, 89–90.

Winter, D.A., Patla, A.E. and Frank, J.S. (1990) Assessment of balance control in humans. *Medical Progress through Technology 16*, 1–2, 31–51.

Ankle Rehabilitation: Key Exercises and Timeline

Fundamental strength work

Plantarflexion

Loop the resistance band around the sole of the foot.
Hold the remainder of the band in the hands.
Point the foot away from the leg. Slowly return to neutral.

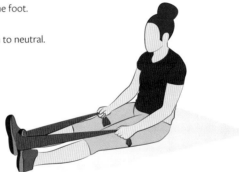

Dorsiflexion

Tie the ends of a resistance band to something sturdy and place the loop around the top of the foot.

Sit back until there is adequate tension in the band.

Pull the foot up towards the shin. Slowly return to neutral.

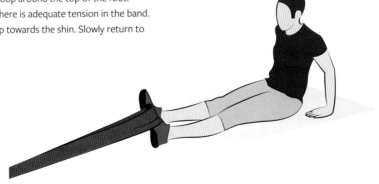

Inversion

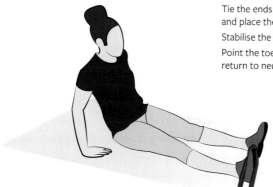

Tie the ends of a resistance band to something sturdy and place the loop around the inside of the foot.

Stabilise the leg with the hands if necessary.

Point the toes inward towards the other foot. Slowly return to neutral.

Eversion

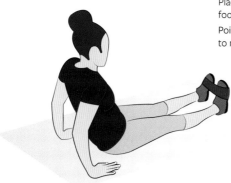

Place the resistance band around the outside of the foot. Loop the band under the opposite foot.

Point the foot out away from the body. Slowly return to neutral.

All the above exercises are carried out seated on the floor or on a chair, with a resistance band that is challenging for the patient.

Progressive strength work

Progressions are listed in order of difficulty from low to high.

Heel raises
Double-leg heel raise

Stand on flat ground with the feet hip-width apart. Use a chair or wall to help stabilise if needed.

Push up on to the balls of the feet as high as you can.

Slowly lower until the heels are on the ground.

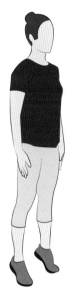

Single-leg heel raise – deficit

Stand on the edge of a stop with only the ball of the left foot in contact. Use a chair or wall to help stabilise if needed.

Push up on to the ball of the left foot as high as you can.

Slowly lower the heel into pain-free range.

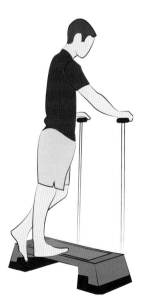

Single-leg heel raise

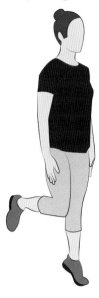

Stand on flat ground with the feet hip-width apart. Use a chair or wall to help stabilise if needed.

Push up on to the ball of the left foot as high as you can.

Slowly lower until the heel is on the ground.

Repeat for the right-hand side.

Single-leg heel raise – weighted

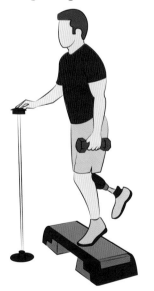

Stand on the edge of a step with only the ball of the left foot in contact. Use a chair or wall to help stabilise if needed.

In the opposite hand, hold a dumbbell or kettlebell that is challenging for you.

Push up on to the ball of the left foot as high as you can.

Slowly lower the heel into pain-free range.

Repeat for the right-hand side.

Step ups
Step up/down

Stand in front of a step with the feet hip-width apart.

Step up on to the step with the left foot and down with the right.

Repeat in reverse for the opposite side.

Begin with a small step and increase the height as progress is made.

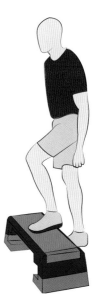

Elevated heel touches

Stand on the floor or on a step with the left foot and the right foot in front.

Slowly lower until the heel of the right foot touches the ground.

Repeat for the right-hand side.

Begin with a small step and increase the height as progress is made.

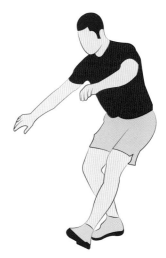

Split squats

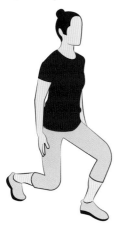

Stand in a split stance with most of your weight on the front leg.

Lower the rear knee towards the ground.

Drive the front leg and hip into standing.

Repeat for the opposite side.

Front-foot elevated split squat

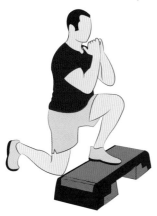

Stand with one foot on a step in front of you.

Lower the hips into a split squat with good posture, allowing the knees to come over the toes.

Drive the hips up into a split stance.

Front-foot elevated split squat – with weight

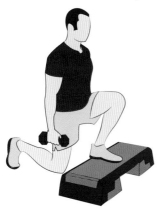

Stand with one foot on a step in front of you, with a dumbbell or kettlebell in one or both hands.

Lower the hips into a split squat with good posture, allowing the knees to come over the toes.

Drive the hips up into a split stance.

Dorsiflexion
Seated dorsiflexion

Sit on a bench with the foot and ankle off the edge.

Place a band through a small weight plate and secure to the foot.

Pull the foot up towards the shin and slowly lower all the way down.

Repeat for the opposite side.

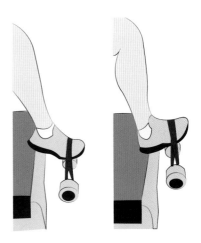

Standing dorsiflexion

Stand with the back against the wall, with the feet about 30 cm from the wall (your bottom will be placed against the wall).

Standing on the heels, point the toes all the way up to the shins and slowly lower until the foot is on the ground.

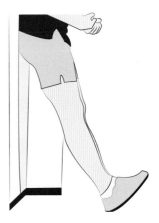

Balance and proprioception

Static balance
Both feet, eyes open

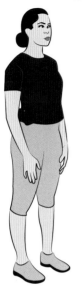

Stand on both feet with arms by your side or across the chest.

Focus on something at eye level. Maintain a good balance.

One foot, eyes open

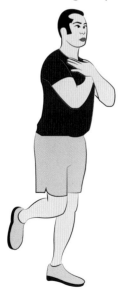

Stand on both feet with arms across the chest.

Bend one knee to 90°.

Focus on something at eye level. Maintain a good balance.

Repeat for the opposite leg.

Both feet, eyes closed

Stand on both feet with arms by your side or across the chest.

Close both eyes.

Maintain a good balance and feel the floor through the feet.

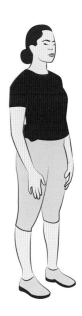

One foot, eyes closed

Stand on both feet with arms across the chest.

Bend one knee to 90°.

Close both eyes and feel the floor through the foot.

Maintain a good balance.

Repeat for the opposite leg.

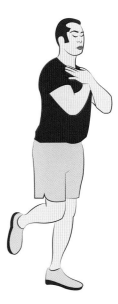

Balance cushion – one foot, eyes open

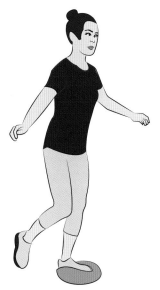

Stand on both feet with arms by your side or across the chest.

Place one foot on the balance cushion and bend the opposite knee to 90°.

Maintain a good balance.

Repeat for the opposite leg.

Balance cushion – one foot, eyes closed

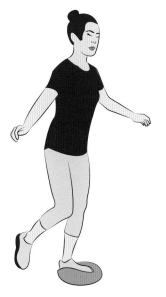

Stand on both feet with arms by your side or across the chest.

Place one foot on the balance cushion and bend the opposite knee to 90°.

Close both eyes and feel the floor through the foot.

Maintain a good balance.

Repeat for the opposite leg.

Dynamic balance
Single-leg Romanian deadlift – assisted

Stand hip-width apart, with both knees slightly bent.

Using the arms out to the sides to aid balance and one hand in contact with a wall or chair, hinge forward at the hips. Allow the non-stance leg to stay in line with the torso.

Drive with the hips to come back to neutral.

Repeat for the opposite side.

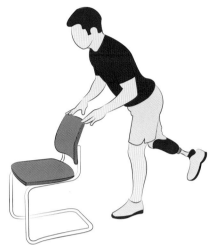

Single-leg Romanian deadlift

Stand hip-width apart, with both knees slightly bent.

Using the arms out to the sides to aid balance, hinge forward at the hips. Allow the non-stance leg to stay in line with the torso.

Drive with the hips to come back to neutral.

Repeat for the opposite side.

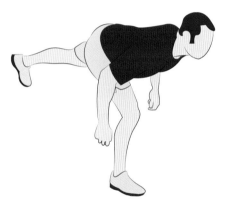

Single-leg Romanian deadlift – weighted

Stand hip-width apart, with both knees slightly bent.

Stand on the left leg and hold the weight in the right hand.

Hinge forward at the hips, allowing the non-stance leg to stay in line with the torso.

Drive with the hips to come back to neutral.

Repeat for the opposite side.

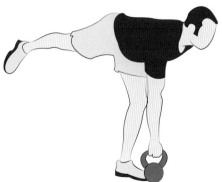

Plyometrics
Double-leg hops – on the spot

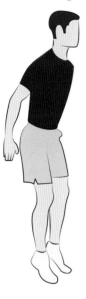

Stand with feet hip-width apart.

Hop up and down, placing the contact of the floor through the balls of the feet.

Only allow the heels to come very close to the floor, around 1–3 cm.

Single-leg hops

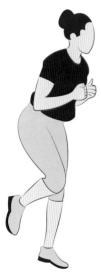

Stand with feet hip-width apart.

Bend the right knee to 90°.

Hop up and down, placing the contact of the floor through the ball of the foot.

Only allow the heel to come very close to the floor, around 1–3 cm.

Single-leg hops – side to side or front to back

Stand with feet hip-width apart.

Bend the right knee to 90°.

Hop forward and back or side to side, placing the contact of the floor through the ball of the foot.

Only allow the heel to come very close to the floor, around 1–3 cm.

Repeat for the opposite side.

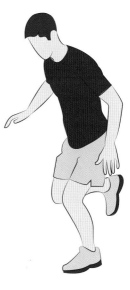

Jump

Stand on a flat surface with the feet hip-width apart.

Bend the knees and hips slightly into a partial squat and explode upwards.

Land on the balls of the feet, allowing the heels to come 1–3 cm off the floor.

Ensure the landing is soft, with the hips and knees slightly bent.

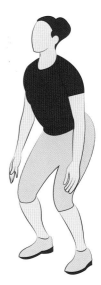

2–1 jump

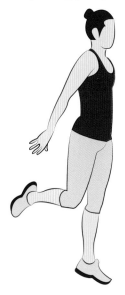

Stand on a flat surface with the feet hip-width apart.

Bend the knees and hips slightly into a partial squat and explode upwards.

Land on the ball of the left foot only, allowing the heel to come 1–3 cm off the floor.

Ensure the landing is soft, with the hips and knees slightly bent.

Repeat for the opposite leg.

Single-leg jump

Stand on a flat surface with the feet hip-width apart.

Bend one knee to 90°.

Bend the knees and hips slightly into a partial squat and explode upwards.

Land on the ball of the foot, allowing the heel to come 1–3 cm off the floor.

Ensure the landing is soft, with the hips and knees slightly bent.

Repeat for the opposite leg.

Depth drop

Stand on a step or a box with the knees hip-width apart.

Have the knees and hips bent very slightly.

Step off the box with the left leg, landing on the balls of the feet, allowing the heels to come 1–3 cm off the floor.

Step up and repeat, landing with the right leg.

Ensure the landing is soft, with the hips and knees slightly bent.

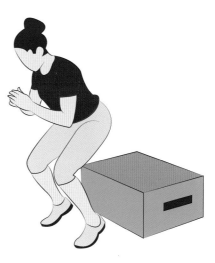

Double-leg clock jumps

Set up either four markers in a diamond or six markers in a hexagon with one in the centre.

With the ankles and knees close together, jump from one marker to the next.

Make sure the landing is soft, with the knees slightly bent.

Ensure you fully stabilise your balance before jumping to the next marker.

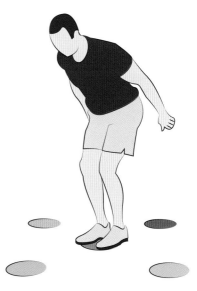

Single-leg clock jumps

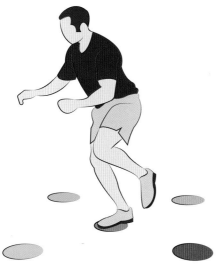

Set up either four markers in a diamond or six markers in a hexagon with one in the centre.

Bend one knee at 90° and jump from one marker to the next.

Make sure the landing is soft, with the knee slightly bent.

Ensure you fully stabilise your balance before jumping to the next marker.

Repeat for the opposite leg.

Flexibility
Tibialis anterior stretch

Kneel on a mat with one or both heels under the sit bones. In this position, you may already feel the stretch running up the shin bones.

To increase the stretch, place the hands behind the feet and lean backwards.

To further increase the stretch, a towel or block may be placed under one or both feet.

Tibialis anterior foam roll

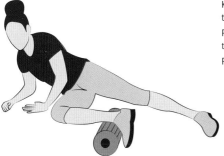

Kneel on a mat with a foam roller under the right tibialis anterior.

Roll the tibialis anterior by flexing and extending at the hip and knee slightly.

Repeat for the opposite side.

Gastrocnemius stretch

Place the ball of the foot on to a step, with the heel in contact with the ground.

Have the stance foot behind, next to or in front of the block. The further forward the stance, the greater the stretch.

Repeat for the opposite side.

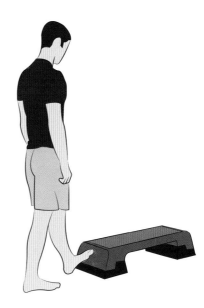

Soleus stretch

Kneel on a mat, with the right foot flat on the floor and kneeling on the left leg.

Push the right knee as far over the toes as possible. You should feel the stretch up the back of the right lower leg.

Swap the position and repeat for the opposite side.

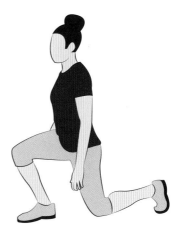

Calf foam roll

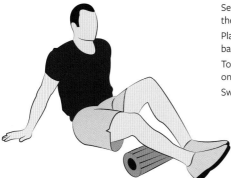

Seated on a flat surface, stabilise with the hands at the sides and the right foot on the floor.

Place the foam roller under the right calf and roll backwards and forwards.

To increase the intensity, the left leg may be placed on top of the right leg.

Swap the position and repeat for the opposite side.

Peroneal foam roll

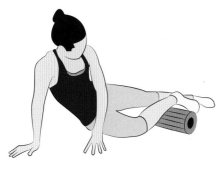

Kneel on a mat with a foam roller under the right peroneal.

Roll the peroneal by flexing and extending slightly at the hip and knee.

Repeat for the opposite side.

Subject Index

Note: illustrations are referenced by page numbers in *italics*

Author Index